Hearing Loss in Musicians

Prevention and Management

The cover picture is from a wonderfully inventive, yet incorrect theory about how the ear hears music. Based on the work of Mr. George Brown in the 1880s, it was argued that in a well-formed pinna, the entire free portion of the cartilage gives a beautifully graduated ascending scale of notes, forming a complete octave from the tragus to the posterior border of the helix—the C major scale. The anti-tragus is responsible for the note E. Mr. Brown maintained that this could be verified by rubbing the various parts of the pinna and listening for the different sounds. (From: "The acoustic potentials of the human auricle," read before the Otological section of the International Medical Congress, 1881.)

Hearing Loss in Musicians

Prevention and Management

Marshall Chasin

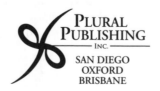

PLURAL
PUBLISHING
INC.

SAN DIEGO
OXFORD
BRISBANE

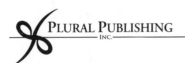

PLURAL PUBLISHING
INC.

5521 Ruffin Road
San Diego, CA 92123

e-mail: info@pluralpublishing.com
Web site: http://www.pluralpublishing.com

49 Bath Street
Abingdon, Oxfordshire OX14 1EA
United Kingdom

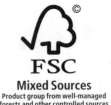

FSC
Mixed Sources
Product group from well-managed
forests and other controlled sources

Cert no. SW-COC-002283
www.fsc.org
© 1996 Forest Stewardship Council

Typeset in 10½/13 Garamond by Flanagan's Publishing Services, Inc
Printed in the United States of America by McNaughton and Gunn, Inc.

For permission to use material from this text, contact us by
Telephone: (866) 758-7251
Fax: (888) 758-7255
e-mail: permissions@pluralpublishing.com

*Every attempt has been made to contact the copyright holders for material originally
printed in another source. If any have been inadvertently overlooked, the publishers
will gladly make the necessary arrangements at the first opportunity.*

Library of Congress Cataloging-in-Publication Data:

Hearing loss in musicians : prevention & management / [edited by] Marshall Chasin.
        p. ; cm.
  Includes bibliographical references and index.
  ISBN-13: 978-1-59756-181-5 (alk. paper)
  ISBN-10: 1-59756-181-9 (alk. paper)
  1.   Deafness, Noise induced—Prevention. 2.   Musicians—Wounds and injuries—
Prevention.   I. Chasin, Marshall.
  [DNLM: 1.   Hearing Loss, Noise-Induced—physiopathology. 2.   Hearing Loss, Noise-
Induced—prevention & control. 3.   Music. 4.   Noise, Occupational—prevention &
control. 5.   Occupational Diseases—prevention & control.   WV 270 H4354 2008]
  RF293.5.H45 2008
  617.8002478—dc22
                                                                              2008024468

Contents

Foreword by Mead Killion   *vii*
Introduction   *ix*
Contributors   *xi*

1 Hearing Loss Prevention for Musicians and Introduction   1
to the Problem
Marshall Chasin

2 Overview of Anatomy and Physiology of the Peripheral   11
Auditory System
Richard J. Salvi, Edward Lobarinas, and Wei Sun

3 The Medical Aspects of Otologic Damage from Noise in Muscians   31
Kenneth Einhorn

4 Tinnitus, Hyperacusis, and Music   41
Richard S. Tyler, Son-A Chang, Pan Tao, Stephanie Gogel, and
Anne K. Gehringer

5 Do Headphones Cause Hearing Loss? Risk of Music Induced   53
Hearing Loss for the Music Consumer
Brian J. Fligor

6 Uniform Hearing Protection for Musicians   63
Patricia A. Niquette

7 Personal In-the-Ear Monitoring: The Audiologist's Role   75
Michael Santucci

8 Room and Stage Acoustics for Optimal Listening and Playing   83
William J. Gastmeier

9 Inexpensive Environmental Modifications   97
Marshall Chasin

10 Hearing Aids and Music   107
Marshall Chasin

11 Cochlear Implants and Music   117
Hugh J. McDermott

12. Music for the Audiologist   129
Marshall Chasin and Doran Hayes

13 Human Performance Approach to Prevention: Occupational   137
Darwinism
John Chong

14 Towards a Functional Hearing Test for Muscians: The Probe   145
Tone Method
Frank A. Russo

Appendixes
  A   Musical Note to Frequency Conversion Chart   153
  B   Six Musicians' Fact Sheets   155

Index   *163*

Foreword

In 1996 Marshall Chasin wrote *Musicians and the Prevention of Hearing Loss* (published by Singular Publishing Group). This was the first book to present and integrate the available knowledge of hearing loss prevention for musicians. It has been more than a decade since the publicaiton of that book and much has been learned. *Hearing Loss in Musicians* is an improved and expanded "second edition" of a book that covers a wide range of topics. Chasin has chosen authors, including himself, who write well about hearing and musicians, with emphasis on the risks to their hearing that musicians face and how they can avoid damage. Chapters cover topics ranging from the differences between noise and music, to basic physiology of hearing and hearing loss, to musician-specific chapters offering practical advice for musicians and their audiologists.

This book is badly needed. I see the problem of music and hearing in my own family. Having worn hearing protection the few times I played piano in a big band, and in my left ear when I practice the violin, I have completely normal hearing through 4 kHz at age 68. My brother, also a musician, has a 55 dB notch at 4 kHz from playing in rock bands and repairing motorcycles (the air hose may have been the main cause of his loss).

Following roughly along the lines of the estimate made by Dan Johnson in his paper, "One Rock Concert = 2½ Year

Aging" (2003), I have estimated that excessive noise or music exposure causes a loss of 1 hair cell for each 16 times overdose. Thus, 160 times the allowable daily maximum costs 10 hair cells. Experience teaches us that a loss of 5 to 10 dB may not be noticed, so it would appear that we have enough redundancy that the effects of losing the first few thousand hair cells may not be noticed. But after that we are on a slippery slope. Even the Rolling Stones concert I attended in Chicago's Soldiers Field produced a steady 104 dBA SPL up in the bleachers, 60 times the allowable exposure after 2 hours. Some heavy metal rock concerts produce 320 times the allowable dose, suggesting a loss of 20 hair cells in 2 hours. Although those 20 hair cells might correspond to only 0.5 dB loss at 4 kHz, losing 10 hair cells a week for 28 years will leave you with only 440 left of your original 15,000 or so.

Many years ago, my engineering mentor, Elmer Carlson, developed a nearly perfect high- fidelity earplug with 15 dB attenuation from 80 Hz to 16 kHz as measured on 10 subjects by Elliott Berger, manager of the EARcal laboratory. Unfortunately, a marketing survey indicated that sales would not be sufficient to justify the cost of introducing this product. The breakthrough came in an unusual fashion. During a performance of Berlioz' "Damnation of Faust," there was a total of nearly 200 singers and Chicago Symphony

Orchestra (CSO) musicians, plus four soloists and the conductor, tightly packed on the old (smaller) Orchestra Hall stage. Bob Lane, one of the viola players, ended up with his head directly in front of the bell of Charlie Vernon's bass trombone. (The CSO trombone section has the reputation of being the only trombone section in the world that makes more noise than the trumpet section, and Vernon is arguably the most powerful trombone player in the business.) At the end of the concert, Bob Swan couldn't hear. A visit to an otolaryngologist confirmed that there was no wax in his ears, but fortunately a course of steroids brought his hearing back "like a teenager" over the next couple of weeks. Nonetheless, it emphasized that there was a danger of hearing damage even for a symphony orchestra musician. A Sound Level Committee was formed, and I was honored to be asked to be a consultant. Three solutions were discussed for those times when the orchestra was playing large, loud pieces: plastic barriers, "buffalo chairs" that partly shielded the player from sounds behind him, and earplugs. When the dust had settled, Etymotic Research obtained a license to manufacture what we named the "Musicians earplugs" because Elmer was too modest to allow us to call them the "Carlson Earplugs."

Over the years, drummers reported that the 15 dB attenuation was fine for classical and jazz playing, but not enough for rock engagements. And viola players reported that 15 dB was a little too much. In response to those requests, we introduced the 25 dB and 9 dB versions of the Musicians earplug. Since custom earmolds are required for the Musicians earplugs, the next step was to develop in cooperation with E-A-R company the one-size-fits-most triple-flange HiFi Earplug with about 20 dB attenuation.

At one time, most of us thought that playing in orchestras or directing a school band was safe. It isn't. I have already reported the normal hearing in the right ear, and the 55 dB music-induced notch in his left ear, measured on Ruben Gonzales, then concertmaster of the CSO. He was a virtuoso soloist playing a powerful Bergonzi violin out over the orchestra as he soloed with orchestras around the world. Another example: Last year when I lectured on hearing protection for some of the Northwestern School of Music students, Prof. Charlie Geyer related to me that after 12 years sitting in the fourth trumpet seat (right next to the percussion) in the Chicago Symphony Orchestra, "It creeps up on you so slowly that you don't notice it, then you find you can't use the telephone on your right ear." Finally, the largest group of musicians with hearing loss is probably high school band directors. We have had an Etymotic booth at the Band Directors Clinic in December in Chicago for many years, and have only met one band director who has been directing school bands for many years who didn't have a hearing loss.

This book is needed and should help prevent music-induced hearing loss among those who bring us one of life's greatest joys.

Mead C. Killion

Reference

Johnson, D. (2003). One rock concert = 2½ year aging. *Spectrum, 20*(1), 6–7.

Introduction

This book about musicians and the prevention of hearing loss brings together both clinical knowledge and research spanning more than three decades of work. Much has been learned and newer technologies are continually becoming available, all for the benefit of ensuring that "what is done today will ensure that the musician will still be able to play and enjoy the music in 30 years." This last phrase is part of the mission statement of the Musicians' Clinics of Canada (2008) and represents a constructive approach to protecting musicians, either by altering their environment, or protecting their hearing directly.

There are several themes that run through this book. One is that any music can be safely played and listened to with good fidelity and quality if it is done correctly. It is more often an issue of presenting the music slightly differently that can make it both safe and enjoyable. Another theme is that a mere 3 dB reduction in intensity effectively cuts the potential damage in half. A reduction of 3 dB is barely noticeable but it can make a large difference.

Hearing Loss in Musicians represents an update of the state of the art in working with musicians. The original text on this topic, *Musicians and the Prevention of Hearing Loss*, is now more than a decade old. A number of "hearing loss prevention practitioners" and researchers have been brought together in this book,

covering the full range of topics and issues that relate to hearing loss prevention for musicians. The book is divided up into three sections—the problem (Chapters 1-5), some solutions (Chapters 6-11), and a section containing a primer on what audiologists need to know about music, occupational aspects of musicians and hearing loss, and future forms of assessment. (Chapters 12-14).

In the problem series of chapters, the history of the problem of hearing loss prevention for musicians is reviewed, followed by a clear yet in-depth overview of the anatomy and physiology of our auditory system. The medical aspects of hearing loss are covered, as are the issues of tinnitus and hyperacusis. It is important to note that the emphasis is not just hearing loss prevention, but almost as importantly, prevention of tinnitus and pitch perception problems. All too often it is tinnitus and pitch perception difficulties that are the issues considered when ending a musical career. The next chapter covers the latest knowledge and advice about the potential for hearing loss from portable and recreational music.

In the solutions series of chapters, uniform attenuation earplugs and personal ear monitor systems are discussed, both of which reduce the sound level at the musician's ear. These chapters are followed by two room acoustics/environmental strategies chapters about how the environment can be improved for better and safer listening. The chapter, Inexpensive Environmental Modifications, is written with the lay person or musician in mind. Chapters in this solutions section also include fitting the hard of hearing musician (or listener) with hearing aids or cochlear implants, and the latest issues and approaches are discussed.

The final series of chapters, 12–14, starts with a primer of some things that audiologists may want to know in order to work with musicians, followed by some unique problems and issues of musicians from an occupational perspective. The final chapter discusses alternative methods of improving the assessment of musicians in order to prevent and treat musicians and those who like to listen to music.

Taken together, these chapters serve as the knowledge basis for the optimal treatment and care for the musician, and for those who are not particularly talented but just like to listen to music (like me).

There are many people to thank, but first and foremost, I would like to thank the authors who graciously agreed to contribute to this book and share with us their knowledge. Special thanks go to my wife Joanne and children, Courtney, Meredith, and Shaun, for their support and putting up with a "preoccupied" husband and father during the work on this book.

The royalties from the sale of this book will go to support educational activities by the Musicians' Clinics of Canada in the prevention of hearing loss among musicians.

Marshall Chasin, AuD.
Editor
Musicians' Clinics of Canada

Reference

Musicians' Clinics of Canada (2008). *Mission statement.* Retrieved November 17, 2008, from http://www.musiciansclinics.com

Contributors

Son-A Chang, MA
Department of Otolaryngology
The University of Iowa
Iowa City, IA
Postgraduate Program of Speech,
    Language, and Hearing Science
Yonsei University, Korea
Chapter 4

**Marshall Chasin, AuD., Aud(C),
    Reg. CASLPO**
Musicians' Clinics of Canada, Toronto,
    Ontario
Adjunct Professor, University of
    Toronto, Department of Linguistics,
    Toronto, Ontario, Canada
Associate Professor, University of
    Western Ontario, School of
    Communication Sciences &
    Disorders, Faculty of Health
    Sciences, London, Ontario, Canada
Chapters 1, 9, 10, and 12

**John Chong, MD, BaSc, MSc, CGPP,
    ARCT**
Musicians' Clinics of Canada
Hamilton, Ontario, Canada
Chapter 13

Kenneth H. Einhorn, MD
Chief, Division of Otolaryngology
Abington Memorial Hospital
Abington, PA
Assistant Professor
Department of Otolaryngology
Temple University
Chapter 3

Brian J. Fligor, ScD
Director of Diagnostic Audiology
Children's Hospital of Boston
Instructor in Otology and Laryngology
Harvard Medical School
Boston, MA
Chapter 5

William J. Gastmeier, MASc, PEng
Principal Engineer
HGC Engineering (Howe Gastmeier
    Chapnik Limited)
Adjunct Professor
University of Waterloo School of
    Architecture
Mississauga, Ontario, Canada
Chapter 8

Anne K. Gehringer, MA, CCC-A
Research Audiologist
University of Iowa Hospitals and Clinics
Iowa City, IA
Chapter 4

Stephanie A. Gogel, MA, CCC-A
Research Audiologist
University of Iowa Hospitals and Clinics
Department of Otolaryngology
Iowa City, IA
Chapter 4

**Doran Hayes, BAM, MSc Aud(C),
    Reg. CASLPO**
Peterborough, Ontario
Canada
Chapter 12

Mead C. Killion, PhD, ScD (hon.)
President, Etymotic Research, Inc.
Adjunct Professor of Audiology
Northwestern University
ScD (Honoray Doctor of Science),
    Wabash College
Crawfordsville, IN
Foreword

Edward Lobarinas, PhD, CCC-A
State University of New York at Buffalo
Center for Hearing and Deafness
Buffalo, NY
Chapter 2

Hugh J. McDermott, PhD
Professor of Auditory Communication
    and Signal Processing
Department of Otolaryngology
The University of Melbourne
East Melbourne, Australia
Chapter 11

Patricia A. Niquette, AuD
Audiologist
Etymotic Research, Inc.
Elk Grove Village, IL
Chapter 6

Tao Pan, MD, PhD
Associate Professor
Department of Otolaryngology
Peking University Third Hospital
Beijing, China
Chapter 11

Frank A. Russo, PhD
Assistant Professor
Ryerson University
Toronto, Ontario, Canada
Chapter 14

Richard Salvi, PhD
Professor, Department of
    Communicative Disorders and
    Sciences, Department of Neurology,
    and Department of Otolaryngology
Director, Center for Hearing and
    Deafness
University at Buffalo
Buffalo, NY
Chapter 2

Michael Santucci, MS, F-AAA
Audiologist/President
Sensaphonics Hearing Conservation, Inc.
http://www.sensaphonics.com
Chicago, IL
Chapter 7

Wei Sun, PhD
Assistant Professor
Department of Communicative
    Disorders and Sciences
Center for Hearing and Deafness
University at Buffalo
Buffalo, NY
Chapter 2

Pan Tao
Department of Otolaryngology Head
    and Neck Surgery
The University of Iowa
Iowa City, IA
Chapter 4

Richard S. Tyler, PhD
Department of Otolaryngology Head
    and Neck Surgery
Department of Communication
    Sciences
The University of Iowa
Iowa City, IA
Chapter 4

1 Hearing Loss Prevention for Musicians and Introduction to the Problem

BY MARSHALL CHASIN

INDUSTRIAL NOISE AND MUSIC

Music and industrial noise have many similarities and some interesting differences. Depending on the musical instrument, the spectral shape and concentration of energy can be quite similar to those of an industrial noise spectrum. This is true of stringed, vocal, brass, and woodwind instruments. It is not true, however, of percussive instruments such as the drums or cymbals—this spectrum is more consistent with the noise spectra found in stamping plants where the sudden percussive sounds yield a broadband spectrum with significant high frequency energy components. However, most industrial noise spectra have their spectral energy based in the lower frequency range with very little energy above 1500 Hz. In contrast, many forms of music can have a broadband spectrum where the higher frequency harmonic structure can be more intense than the lower frequency fundamental energy. Because of this spectral difference, the nature of the hearing loss resulting from the music exposure can be subtly different from exposure to an equivalent intensity noise spectrum. This however, is not always the case, and it is not uncommon to find that a music spectrum and an industrial noise spectrum have similar shapes and intensities. In many cases, only the client history can provide clues to the etiology of the hearing loss.

There can also be substantial intensity differences both in terms of the overall intensities and the dynamic ranges (difference between the most and least intense components). Instrumental music has a dynamic range on the order of 100 dB with brush sounds on the drum typically being the least intense and amplified and percussive music being the most intense. Using modern hearing aid terminology, instrumental music can have a modulation depth of 100 dB (and a modulation rate of up to 100 Hz)—meaning the dynamic range can be around 100 dB and it can vary in intensity up to 100 times per second. Vocal music can have modulation rates around 2 to 10 Hz with the bulk of the singing being between 4 and 6 Hz. (Chung, 2004). In contrast, industrial noise (and most noise sources) has a very low modulation rate (<2 Hz) and an almost nonexistent modulation depth (i.e., very little intensity difference between the most intense and least intense noise components). Industrial noise however can have more sustained high intensity periods than are typically found with music. Music tends to have greater dynamics with short periods of relative quiet followed by periods of greater intensity.

KEY POINT

Differences between music and noise are more in the realm of intensity dynamic ranges and in the temporal characteristics rather than the spectral shape or peak intensity measures.

The differences between music and noise are therefore more in the realm of intensity dynamic ranges and in the temporal characteristics rather than the spectral shape or peak intensity measures. Wagner's "Ring Cycle" (Camp & Horstman, 1992) has levels similar to the most intense industrial environments, and many forms of jazz and folk music have levels similar to that of a busy, but quiet, office environment. Table 1-1, adapted from Camp and Horstman (1992, based on what is considered to be the most intense classical music), shows intensities for some instruments during the most intense movement ("Gotterdammerung").

Table 1-2 (adapted from Chasin, 2006) shows measurements of a wide range of musical instruments measured in the horizontal plane at a distance of 3 meters. All measurements were performed in a typical musical environment for that particular instrument and are measured in dBA.

Table 1–1. Measurements of peak SPL taken during the most intense movement of the Wagner's Ring Cycle, considered to be the most intense piece of classical music.

Instrument	Peak Levels (dB SPL)
French horn	107
Bassoon	102
Trombone	108
Tuba	110
Trumpet	111
Violin	109
Clarinet	108
Percussion	>120

Note. Adapted from "Musician Sound Exposure during Performance of Wagner's 'Ring Cycle'," by J. E. Camp and S. W. Horstman, 1992, *Medical Problems of Performing Artists, 7*(2), pp. 37–39. Adapted with permission.

FACTORS AFFECTING HEARING LOSS

PTS and TTS

Understandably, many of the seminal studies on the effects of noise exposure (and by extension, music exposure) are either based on animal models where a permanent threshold shift (PTS) has been created, or on humans in well-controlled laboratory-based experiments where a temporary threshold shift (TTS) has been created. As the name suggests, TTS typically resolves within 16 to 18 hours, but tinnitus may last several days. TTS, like PTS, typically occurs one half octave above the offending stimulus frequency,

Table 1-2. Unless otherwise specified (e.g., "near left ear"), all measurements were taken at 3 meters for a large number of musicians (inner two quartiles) using differing styles of playing and different instruments.

Musical instruments at 3 meters (at 0° azimuth)	dBA
Normal piano practice	60–90
Loud piano practice	70–105
Keyboards (electric)	60–110
Vocalist	70–85
Chamber music (classical)	70–92
Violin/viola (near left ear)	85–105
Violin/viola	80–90
Cello	80–104
Acoustic bass	70–94
Clarinet	68–82
Oboe	74–102
Saxophone	75–110
Flute (near right ear)	98–114
Flute	92–105
Piccolo (near right ear)	102–118
Piccolo	96–112[1]
French horn	92–104
Trombone	90–106
Trumpet	88–108
Tympani and bass drum	74–94
Percussion (at left ear near high hat)	68–94; peak 125 dB SPL
Amplified guitar (using in-ear monitoring)	100–106
Amplified guitar (using wedge loudspeaker monitoring)	105–112
Symphonic music	86–102
Amplified rock music	102–108
MP-3 player (volume 6/10)	94
MP-3 player (full-on volume)	105

[1]With a peak level of 126 dB SPL, piccolo players are banned from my office!

Note. From "How Loud Is that Musical Instrument?" by M Chasin, 2006, *Hearing Review, 13*(3), p. 26. Used with permission.

and in the unprotected ear the offending frequency is near the natural ear outer canal resonance, which is between 2700 and 3000. TTS and PTS therefore manifest themselves first in the 3000 to 6000 Hz region, although it is not unusual to find a "noise notch" in the audiogram up to 8000 Hz (especially for violins and picollo players). Mills et al. (1983) found that for very low frequency stimuli (below 500 Hz), the TTS would be in the 300 to 750 Hz region, regardless of the exact stimulus frequency.

In the mid-1960s the Committee on Hearing and Bioacoustics (CHABA) tried to establish a predictive relationship between TTS and PTS. They argued that "If any single band exceeds the damage-risk contour specified, the noise can be considered as potentially unsafe" (Kryter, Ward, Miller, & Eldredge, 1966). This research led to the development of a series of damage risk criteria (DRC). If the measured noise levels did not achieve the DRC contour, then it was not damaging. At that time, several assumptions were made: (a) regular "quiet periods" would reduce the risk, and (b) recovery from TTS was only related to the magnitude of the stimulus.

The CHABA report discusses the "on fraction rule" as a rule that " . . . predicts that when the noise is on for half of the total period of exposure, the amount of TTS would be one-half of that which would have been predicted if the noise had been continuous" (Melnick, 1991, p. 150). That is, damage can be mitigated by intermittency. Melnick (1991) also showed that the recovery from TTS was related to both the magnitude and the duration of the exposure.

A decade later, Dixon Ward (Ward, Cushing, & Burns, 1976), who was one of the architects of the CHABA report, developed upper limits of "effective quiet" —levels that would produce no TTS— and these were significantly less than those stated by CHABA. The quiet periods would serve to reduce the amount of predicted damage. The estimates of effective quiet are given in Table 1-3,

Table 1-3. Estimates of "effective quiet" (Ward, Cushing, & Burns., 1976) and a comparison of levels from the location in a classical orchestra of three instrument sections while they were not playing.

Frequency (Hz)	Effective Quiet (dB SPL)	Clarinet (dB SPL)	Violin (dB SPL)	Trumpet (dB SPL)
250	77	72–82	75–84	75–98
500	76	73–84	75–87	76–98
1000	69	69–81	71–78	70–87
2000	68	66–74	70–74	66–77
4000	65	56–62	59–65	60–67
Broadband	76 dBA			

Note. From *Musicians and the Prevention of Hearing Loss* (1st ed., p. 27), by M. Chasin, 1996, Clifton Park, NY: Delmar Learning. Reprinted with permission of Delmar Learning, a division of Thomson Learning.

along with intensity ranges measured in three classical instrument sections while the musicians were *not* playing. Note that all three instrument groups exceeded the effective quiet levels even when not playing. It should be noted that these are not *critical levels*, which are octave band levels that would cause *5 dB of TTS* after 16 hours of exposure. Once corrected for the difference in definition, the Ward et al. (1976) data are consistent with the later work of Mills et al. (1979), which uses critical levels.

PTS and TTS Revisited

While it would be tempting to conclude that someone who is very susceptible to TTS in a well-controlled study would also be someone who is more susceptible to PTS, there is no evidence to support this. At most, one could say that TTS is a necessary precursor to PTS. One of the reasons is that PTS and TTS may have different physiological mechanisms.

Henderson et al. (2006) argued that there are two possible mechanisms of TTS and that these are probably not identical to those of PTS (cell death due to necrosis or apoptosis), although there may be some overlap. When TTS occurs, the tips of the outer hair cells can become disconnected from the tectorial membrane and result in a hearing loss. However, there is a period of time that the hair cells can become reconnected to the tectorial membrane, thereby reestablishing the previous hearing levels. This is the most probable explanation for TTS. TTS may also be brought about by glutamate ototoxicity. Glutamate is an excitatory neurotransmitter substance that occurs in the synapse between the inner hair cells and the VIII auditory nerve. With high levels of glutamate brought about by high levels of noise, this substance can become ototoxic and cause the postsynaptic cells to swell. This is thought to be a temporary condition. Using a glutamate blocker will minimize TTS in some experimental situations.

KEY POINT

The relationship between PTS and TTS are not well defined, but TTS is a necessary precursor to PTS.

PTS AND MODELS

Between 1968 and 1973 there were a number of large scale field studies relating to the relationship between noise exposure and PTS. (Baughn, 1973; Lempert & Henderson, 1973; Passchier-Vermeer, 1968, 1971; Robinson, 1968, 1971). The Passchier-Vermeer, Robinson, and Baughn studies served as the basis of the 1973 United States Environmental Protection Agency's (EPA) Criteria Document. These studies noted very little PTS for long-term exposure (40 years) to 8-hour work day exposures of 85 dBA or less, averaged at 500 Hz, 1000 Hz, and 2000 Hz. There was poor predictive ability for 3000 Hz and 4000 Hz hearing acuity. The Lempert and Henderson (1973) study formed the basis of the National Institute for Occupational Safety and Health (NIOSH) model. A more recent model is the one developed by the International Organization for Standardization (ISO) R-1999 (1990), which, for the most part, is consistent with previous models and is " . . . sufficiently accurate to support the needs of most regulators, administrators, and others who

Table 1-4. Five models with predicted PTS at three exposure levels. Note that exposure levels of 85 dBA will still result in some PTS.

	Passchier-Vermeer	Robinson	Baughn	NIOSH	ISO R-1999
85 dBA	8	6	9	5	6
90 dBA	15	12	14	11	11
95 dBA	23	18	17	20	21

Note. From *Musicians and the Prevention of Hearing Loss* (1st ed.), by M. Chasin, 1996, Clifton Park, NY: Delmar Learning. Reprinted with permission of Delmar Learning, a division of Thomson Learning.

need rough predictions on the effects of noise on groups of workers" (Johnson, 1991, p. 174). Table 1-4 compares the predicted PTS at 4000 Hz for three exposure levels, in five models. Exposure levels as quiet as 85 dBA are predicted to still cause a small, but measurable, PTS.

EXCHANGE RATES

The CHABA DRCs specify contours of equal risk for PTS given a specified exposure level *and* exposure time. The relationship between exposure level and time exposed is called the exchange rate. A 3 dB exchange rate (or 3 dB-rule) means that the exposure is identical if a person is exposed at a level 3 dB more intense but for half the time. That is, there is a *trade-off* or *exchange* between intensity and duration. A 5 dB exchange rate, for example, would mean that a 90 dBA exposure for 40 hours a week is equivalent to a 95 dBA exposure for only 20 hours. Correspondences can be derived using simple algebra—85 dBA for 40 hours a week = 88 dBA for 20 hours a week = 91 dBA for 10 hours a week, and so on.

This relationship appears to be valid for exposures up to about 115 dBA. There is a paucity of data to support such a relationship above this point.

Although there has been some historical debate about whether the 3 dB or the 5 dB exchange rate is most appropriate, Embleton (1995) concluded that "the scientific evidence is that 3 dB is probably the most reasonable exchange rate for daily noise exposure" (p. 18). It should be noted that "exchange rates" are only meant to summarize the data. Ward (1982) stated that the effects of noise exposure are caused by dosage, not merely sound level. Some jurisdictions around the world still use the 5 dB exchange rate, but there is no science supporting this decision. Further discussion on DRCs and exchange rates can be found in Chapter 6.

KEY POINT

Although there has been some historical debate about whether the 3 dB or the 5 dB exchange rate is most appropriate, most of the evidence points to the 3 dB exchange rate.

AUDIOMETRIC ASYMMETRIES

A hallmark of industrial noise exposure is a symmetrical hearing loss on the audiogram (with a "typical" noise notch in the 3000 Hz–6000 Hz region; Alberti, 1982). The two reasons for this symmetry are that (a) most industrial noise is concentrated in the lower frequency region and (b) industrial workers frequently find themselves in reverberant environments. Because low frequency sounds have long wavelengths, the head and body do not represent a shadow for the noise. A noise source emanating from the right side of the worker can be just as intense at the left ear as the right ear. This is exacerbated by the environmental reverberation, where reflected noise bounces off walls and other obstructions with minimal loss of energy. The result is the sound field on one side of the head is similar to that on the other side regardless of where the noise initially emanated from.

KEY POINT

Because of the significant higher frequency energy content of music, coupled with performing and listening in relatively nonreverberant environments, audiometric asymmetries may be found.

In contrast, music has significant mid- and high frequency energy components and is typically played or heard in relatively nonreverberant environments. The shorter wavelengths found in the treble notes undergo significant attenuation from one side of the body to the other—head and body baffle effects. And with the relative lack of reverberation, reflected echoes are of lower intensity. A violinist who holds his instrument near the left ear will receive a much higher sound level at the left ear than the right ear for the above reasons. Slight audiometric asymmetries are therefore frequently found. These asymmetries may amount to up to 25 dB (e.g., a drummer with the high-hat cymbal near the left ear), but larger asymmetries are not typical of music exposure and should be investigated in order to rule out retrocochlear pathologies. Depending on one's clinical protocols, all asymmetries should be investigated, even though some of them may be explained in terms of head shadow and body baffle effects.

SUMMARY

The differences between music and noise are more in the realm of intensity dynamic ranges and in the temporal characteristics rather than the spectral shape or peak intensity measures. In many instances music has significantly more high frequency energy content, but this is not always the case. It is this high frequency energy content (coupled with a relatively nonreverberant environment) that can result in audiometric asymmetries with musicians.

In 1966, the Committee on Hearing and Bioacoustics (CHABA) tried to establish a predictive relationship between TTS and PTS. These resulted in damage risk criteria (DRC), but despite the common use of these "equal exposure" contours, they are based on some questionable assumptions. PTS and TTS are not always corellated, and the most that can be said is that one cannot have PTS from long-term noise or music exposure without first having TTS. This may be related, in part, to differing mechanisms underlying PTS and TTS.

Although there has been some historical debate about whether the 3 dB or the 5 dB exchange rate is most appropriate, Embleton (1995) concluded that "the scientific evidence is that 3 dB is probably the most reasonable exchange rate for daily noise exposure" (p. 18).

Acknowledgement. Some of the material used in this chapter was adapted with permission from *Musicians and the Prevention of Hearing Loss* (1st ed.), by M. Chasin, 1996, published by Delmar Learning, a division of Thomson Learning.

REFERENCES

Alberti, P. W. (Ed.). (1982). *Personal hearing protection in industry*. New York: Raven Press.

Baughn, W. L. (1973). *Relation between daily noise exposure and hearing loss as based on the evaluation of 6835 industrial noise exposure cases* (TR AMRL-TR-73-53, AD 767 204). Dayton, OH: Aerospace Medical Research Laboratory, Wright-Patterson Air Force Base.

Camp, J. E., & Horstman, S. W. (1992). Musician sound exposure during performance of Wagner's Ring Cycle., *Medical Problems of Performing Artists*, 7(2), 37–39.

Chasin, M. (2006). How loud is that musical instrument? *Hearing Review*, 13(3), 26.

Chung, K. (2004). Challenges and recent developments in hearing aids. Part I. Speech understanding in noise, microphone technologies and noise reduction algorithms. *Trends in Amplification*, 8(3), 83–124.

Embleton, T. (1995). Upper limits on noise in the workplace. Report by the International Institute of Noise Control Engineering Working Party, *Canadian Acoustics*, 23(2), 11-20.

Henderson, D., Bielefeld, E., Carney Harris, K., & Hu, B. H. (2006). The role of oxidative stress in noise-induced hearing loss. *Ear and Hearing*, 27(1), 1–19.

International Organization for Standardization. (1990). *Acoustics—Determination of occupational noise exposure and estimation of noise-induced hearing impairment* (2nd ed.). International Standards Organization ISO 1999. Geneva, Switzerland: Author.

Johnson, D. L. (1991). Field studies: Industrial exposures. *Journal of the Acoustical Society of America*, 90(1), 170–174.

Kryter, K. D., Ward, W. D., Miller, J. D., & Eldredge, D. H. (1966). Hazardous exposures to intermittent and steady-state noise. *Journal of the Acoustical Society of America*, 39, 451–464.

Lempert, B. L., & Henderson, T. L. (1973). NIOSH survey of occupational noise and hearing: 1968 to 1972 (TR 86). Washington, DC: U.S. Department of Health, Education and Welfare, National Institute for Occupational Safety and Health.

Melnick, W. (1991). Human temporary threshold shift (TTS) and damage risk. *Journal of the Acoustical Society of America*, 90(1), 147–154.

Mills, J. H., Gilbert, R. M., & Adkins, W. Y. (1979). Temporary threshold shifts in humans exposed to octave bands of noise for 16 to 24 hours. *Journal of the Acoustical Society of America*, 65(5), 1238–1248.

Mills, J. H., Osguthorpe, J. D., Burdick, C. K., Patterson, J. H., & Mozo, B. (1983). Temporary threshold shifts produced by exposure to low-frequency noises. *Journal of the Acoustical Society of America*, 73, 918–923.

Passchier-Vermeer, W. (1968). *Hearing loss due to exposure to steady-state broadband noise* (Rep. No. 35). Amsterdam, The Netherlands: Institute for Public Health Engineering.

Passchier-Vermeer, W. (1971). Steady-state and fluctuating noise: Its effects on the hearing of people. In D. W. Robinson (Ed.), *Occupational hearing loss* (pp. 15–33). New York: Academic Press.

Robinson, D. W. (1968). *The relationship between hearing loss and noise exposure.* (Aero Rep. Ae32). Teddington, England: National Physical Laboratory.

Robinson, D. W. (1971). Estimating the risk of hearing loss due to continuous noise. In D. W. Robinson (Ed.), *Occupational hear-ing loss* (pp. 43–62). New York: Academic Press.

Ward, W. D. (1982). Summation of international symposium on hearing protection in industry. In P. A. Alberti (Ed.), *Personal hearing protection in industry* (pp. 577–592). New York: Raven Press.

Ward, W. D., Cushing, E. M., & Burns, E. M. (1976). Effective quiet and moderate TTS: Implications for noise exposure standards. *Journal of the Acoustical Society of America, 59,* 160–165.

2 Overview of Anatomy and Physiology of the Peripheral Auditory System

BY RICHARD J. SALVI,
EDWARD LOBARINAS, AND WEI SUN

Musicians possess a remarkable array of instruments and vocal styles that can appeal to diverse musical interests ranging from classical and operatic on the one hand to jazz, rock, and rap at the other end of the continuum. Regardless of the musical proclivity of the listener, the melodies, consisting of sound waves, must be transferred from the external ear through the middle ear and into the cochlea, where the mechanical vibrations are transduced into a complex pattern of neural activity (Figure 2–1 a, b, c; Ades & Engstrom, 1974). The neural activity in the cochlea is then relayed on to a series of auditory nuclei in the brainstem, midbrain, auditory cortex (Figure 2–1d), as well as other neural centers in the brain where the sounds are interpreted and imbued with meaning and emotion. This chapter will review some of the important features of the peripheral auditory system that play an important role in coding the frequency (related to pitch perception) and intensity (related to loudness perception) of simple and complex sounds. Figure 2–1a shows the basic elements of the auditory pathway—namely the external ear, the middle ear, the inner ear or cochlea, and the central auditory pathway.

EXTERNAL EAR

The only visible part of the auditory pathway is the external ear. The large, crescent-shaped auricle is composed of a cartilaginous understructure that gives it shape as well as flexibility. A cavity in the auricle is present near the entrance of the ear canal (external auditory canal or meatus). The external auditory canal, which projects medially and anteriorly, terminates at the tympanic membrane, a thin, cone-shaped sheet of tissue.

The main function of the external ear is to collect and funnel sound towards the tympanic membrane. The physical dimensions of the pinna, concha, and external auditory meatus largely determine its acoustic properties. The external ear canal behaves like a tube that is closed at one end. The resonant frequency (Fr) of such a tube is predicted to be 3269 Hz,

11

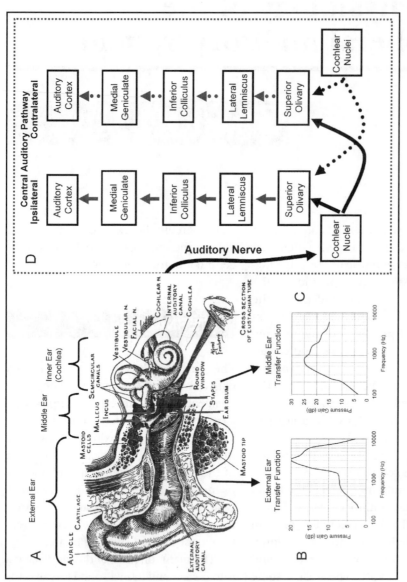

Figure 2–1. (**A**) Anatomy of the external ear, middle ear, cochlea, and cochlear nerve. *Note.* Adapted from "Anatomy of the Inner Ear," by H. W. Ades and H. Engstrom, 1974, in W. D. Keidel and W. D. Neff (Eds.), *Handbook of Sensory Neurology* (Vol. V[1]), p . 126), New York: Springer Verlag. Used with permission. (**B**) External ear transfer function of humans. *Note.* Adapted from "Transformation of Sound Pressure Level from the Free Field to the Eardrum in the Horizontal Plane," by E. A. G. Shaw, 1974 *Journal of the Acoustical Society of America, 56*(6), pp. 1848–1861. Used with permission. (**C**) Middle ear transfer function of the cat. *Note.* Adapted from "Sound Pressures in the Basal Turn of the Cat Cochlea," by V. Nedzelnitsky, 1980, *Journal of the Acoustical Society of America, 68*(6), pp. 1676–1689. Used with permission. (**D**) Highly simplified block diagram of the central auditory pathway. The first major interaural connection between the ipsilateral and contralateral (dashed line) auditory pathways occurs at the level of the cochlear nuclei-superior olivary complex; however, extensive interaural connections exist at higher levels.

where $Fr = c/4$ L, c is the speed of sound (34,000 cm/s), and L is the length of the ear canal, 2.6 cm.

By placing a probe tube microphone near the tympanic membrane and comparing the sound level near the tympanic membrane to the sound field, one can calculate the sound amplification provided by the external ear at different frequencies, that is, the external ear transfer function (E. A. G. Shaw, 1974). Measurements show that the external ear acts like a bandpass amplifier increasing the sound intensity by nearly 20 dB for frequencies near 3000 Hz. In contrast, frequencies below 400 Hz and above 9000 Hz are amplified by 5 dB or less.

KEY POINT

The large increase in sound pressure provided by the external ear in the 3000 Hz region may be one reason why noise-induced hearing loss often begins near 3000 to 4000 Hz.

MIDDLE EAR

Behind the tympanic membrane lies the middle ear space, which is filled with air (see Figure 2–1a). The air within the middle ear communicates with the external environment through the eustachian tube, a narrow, membranous duct that connects with the oral cavity. Under normal conditions, the eustachian tube is open allowing the air pressure behind the tympanic membrane to equilibrate with the ambient air pressure in front of the tympanic membrane. However, when the eustachian tube is blocked due to an infection, the air pressure in the middle ear space will no longer be able to rise or fall with changes in environmental pressure, for example, when airplane cabin pressure changes during takeoff and landing. If the eustachian tube is blocked and the ambient pressure increases, the tympanic membrane will be pushed inward, creating an uncomfortable or painful sensation.

The three middle ear ossicles, consisting of malleus, incus, and stapes, form a series of interconnected bones that couple the tympanic membrane to the fluid-filled inner ear (see Figure 2–1a). At this stage, the vibrations in air will be transferred via the mechanical vibrations of the ossicles. One long arm of the malleus is attached to the tympanic membrane, whereas the other projects medially where a ligament connects the head of the malleus to the body of the incus. The long arm of the incus is attached to the head of the stapes by another ligament. Two struts of bone branch off from the head of the stapes, forming an arch, and attach to the ends of the stapes footplate that lies within the oval window of the fluid-filled cochlea (inner ear). The footplate of the stapes is held within the oval window by a flexible ring of cartilage that allows the footplate to move in and out like a piston. At this stage, the mechanical vibrations of the ossicles will be transferred into fluid motion within the cochlea.

When sound strikes water, the large impedance gradient at the air-water interface causes roughly 99.9% of the energy in the sound wave to bounce back into air; only 0.1% is absorbed into the fluid-filled cochlea. This is roughly equivalent to a 30 dB loss ($10\log10^{-3}$) in pressure when sound moves from air into water. The middle ear overcomes this energy loss by acting as pressure amplifier. The pressure amplification occurs in two ways. First, the area of the tympanic membrane that collects sound is approximately 17 times larger than the area of the stapes footplate that pushes on the fluids in the inner ear. Consequently, the pressure seen by the cochlear fluids behind the stapes is roughly 17 times higher than the pressure at the tympanic membrane (a good analogy is to consider the pressure amplification that occurs between the insole of a high-heeled shoe and the tip of the high heel). This 17 times pressure amplification translates into roughly a 25 dB increase in sound pressure. The second pressure amplification system arises from the fact that the malleus is roughly 1.7 times longer than the incus or a 4.6 dB increase in pressure (This is analogous to lifting a heavy object by placing a heavy rod over a fulcrum and applying pressure to the long arm of the rod.).

KEY POINT

The middle ear acts as a pressure amplification system that restores the loss in pressure that normally would occur when sound is transmitted from air into the fluid-filled cochlea. Damage to the middle ear causes a conductive hearing loss.

COCHLEA (INNER EAR)

The cochlea is contained in a snail-shaped bony capsule that contains three parallel, fluid-filled compartments that spiral around the modiolus from the basal turn towards the apex (Figure 2–2a). The stapes inserts into the oval window near the base of the cochlea. Scala vestibuli, which lies directly behind the oval window, is filled with perilymph that has a fluid composition similar to cerebrospinal fluid, specifically high in sodium (~150 mM) and low in potassium (~3 mM) (Bosher & Warren, 1968). Scala vestibuli extends longitudinally towards the apex of the cochlea where a small opening, the helicotrema, provides a passageway into scala tympani. Scala tympani, which is also filled with perilymph, extends longitudinally from the apex towards the base of the cochlea where it terminates at the round window membrane. The round window membrane is oriented approximately perpendicularly to the oval window. If a radial cross section is taken through a segment of the cochlea (Figure 2–2b), a third fluid-filled chamber, scala media, is seen lying between scala vestibuli and scala tympani. Scala media is filled with endolymph, a unique fluid with a high concentration of potassium (~160 mM) and a relatively low concentration of sodium (~1.6 mM). The concentration of chloride in scala media is similar to that in perilymph (~120–130 mM). The radial cross section shows scala media sandwiched between scala vestibuli and scala tympani (Figure 2–2b). The stria vascularis and spiral ligament form the lateral wall of scala media. Scala media is separated from scala vestibuli by Reissner's membrane (Figure 2–2c). The fluid in scala media is separated from scala tympani by the reticular lamina, a boundary formed by tight cell junctions near the apical surfaces of the cells facing the endolymphatic space. The perilymph in scala tympani passes through the basilar membrane and bathes the cells beneath the reticular lamina.

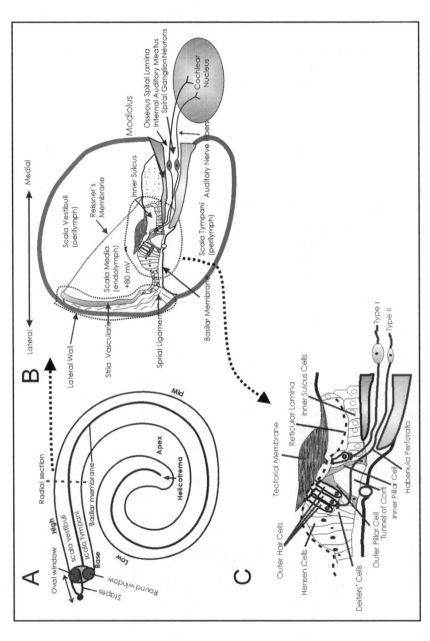

Figure 2–2. **(A)** Schematic showing the snail-shaped cochlea partially uncoiled to show its longitudinal extent. **(B)** Schematic showing a radial cross section (see Figure 2–1b) through a turn of the cochlea. Each turn of the cochlea contains three fluid-filled compartments, scala vestibuli and scala tympani, both filled with perilymph, and scala media, filled with endolymph. The organ of Corti [see the dotted line and arrow pointing to panel (C)] contains the sensory hair cells that convert sound into neural activity. *Note.* Redrawn from *What's New*, No. 199, by B. J. Melloni, 1957, North Chicago, IL: Abbott Laboratories. Used with permission. **(C)** Schematic showing the inner hair cells and outer hair cells and type I and type II neurons in the organ of Corti. *Note.* Redrawn from *Audiology: The Fundamentals* (p. 63), by F. H. Bess and L. E. Humes, 1990, Baltimore: Williams and Wilkins. Used with permission.

Organ of Corti

The organ of Corti containing the sensory hair cells lies on the basilar membrane; the organ of Corti extends medially from the modiolus towards the spiral ligament on the lateral wall (see Figure 2–2b, dashed line). The inner and outer pillar cells form a triangular fluid space in the organ of Corti. The feet of the pillar cells rest on the basilar membrane and the heads of the pillar cells are joined together near the reticular lamina. The three outer hair cell (OHC) rows are located lateral to the outer pillar cells. The base of each OHC rests in a cuplike depression in the Deiters cell, and the apical surface of each OHC is located at the reticular lamina facing scala media. The lateral wall of the OHC is surrounded by fluid spaces. A band of Hensen cells is located lateral to the OHCs. A single row of inner hair cells (IHCs) is located just medial to the inner pillar cells. The supporting cells in the inner sulcus are located medial to the IHCs. The tectorial membrane is an acellular, gelatinous-like structure that is attached at inner sulcus; the tectorial membrane extends laterally over the organ of Corti.

Inner and Outer Hair Cells

The cell bodies of the IHCs and OHCs differ in shape (Figure 2–3). The OHCs are cylindrically shaped and the IHCs are pear-shaped (Figure 2–3b). The nucleus is located near the base of the hair cell and a thickened cuticular plate is located at the apical pole. Stereocilia bundles protrude from the cuticular plate on the apical surface of IHCs and OHCs (Figure 2–3b). Several parallel rows of stereocilia

emerge from the cuticular plate of each hair cell. The stereocilia form a W-shaped bundle on the OHCs, whereas those on the IHCs form a gently curving arc (Figure 2–3a). The heights of the IHC and OHC stereocilia are graded in length (Figure 2–3b). The rows of stereocilia form a staircase pattern; the tallest row of stereocilia is closest to the lateral wall and the shortest row is closest to the modiolus. Each stereocilium contains actin, a structural protein that provides structural rigidity. However, as the root of each stereocilium enters the cuticular plate it narrows, providing a point around which the stereocilium pivots. The rigid stereocilia are joined together by side links that cause the stereocilia bundle to move as a unit, pivoting around the narrow rootlet of the stereocilium.

Transduction

The conversion of sound vibration into neural activity is believed to occur by opening a mechanically gated transduction (ion) channel located near the tip of the stereocilium. The transduction channel is connected to a tip link attached to the side of the taller, neighboring stereocilium. When the stereocilia bundle is deflected in the direction of the tallest row of stereocilia, tension is applied to the tip link and the applied force mechanically pulls the transduction channel open, allowing ions to flow through the stereocilia (Hudspeth, 1992). When the bundle is deflected in the opposite direction towards the shortest row of stereocilia, the tension on the tip link is minimal, allowing the transduction channel to close. When the transduction channel is gated open by sound, potassium ions flow into

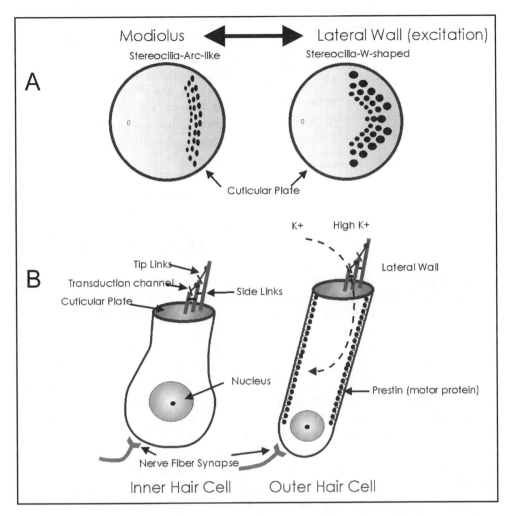

Figure 2–3. (**A**) Apical surface of inner hair cell (*left*) and outer hair cell (*right*) showing arrangement of stereocilia bundle. The stereocilia bundle is arranged in a gently curving arc on inner hair cell and in W- or U-shaped pattern on outer hair cell. (**B**) Radial view showing pear-shaped cell body of inner hair cell and cylindrical shape of outer hair cell. *Note.* Redrawn from *Bases of Hearing Science* (3rd ed., p. 144), by J. D. Durrant and J. H. Lovrinic, 1995, Baltimore: Williams and Wilkins. Used with permission.

the hair cell; this causes the hair cell to depolarize from a resting potential of approximately –60 mV. Two factors promote the influx of potassium. First, there is a large voltage gradient (~140 mV) between the endolymph (+80 mV) and the inside of the hair cell (–60 mV). Second, there is a large potassium concentration gradient between endolymph (~160 mM) and the inside of the hair cell (~5 mM). Consequently, when the transduction channel is open, potassium will flow down its concentration and electrical gradient into the hair cell.

<table>
<tr><td>

KEY POINT

Sound is converted into neural activity by the hair cells. The sound-induced deflection of the stereocilia bundle alters the flow of potassium ions into the hair cells, resulting in a receptor potential.

</td></tr>
</table>

Cochlear Mechanics

Sound-induced movement of the stapes results in pressure fluctuations in the cochlear fluids. Because the cochlear fluids are incompressible, the pressure fluctuations are transmitted virtually instantaneously along the entire basilar membrane from base to apex. Although the pressure is applied instantaneously along the entire basilar membrane, the basilar membrane vibrations appear to travel from the base towards the apex (Bekesy, 1960). The traveling wave vibration pattern arises from the impedance gradient along the length of the basilar membrane. The impedance of each point along the membrane is frequency dependent. The impedance is determined by the mass and stiffness at each point along the basilar membrane. The stiffness of the basilar membrane is greatest near the base and progressively decreases moving towards the apex. On the other hand, the mass of the basilar membrane is greatest near the apex and decreases towards the base. The low mass and high stiffness allow the base to respond sooner to the applied pressure than the apex, which has a lower stiffness and higher mass. The motion of the basilar membrane is opposed by the viscous fluid drag of the perilymph and endolymph, which acts as a resistive element that tends to damp out the energy in the traveling wave.

The point on the basilar membrane that has the lowest impedance at a particular frequency will produce the largest vibration amplitude. Figure 2–4 shows the traveling wave amplitude displacement (nm) as a function of distance along the basilar membrane for 8000 Hz, 4000 Hz, and 200 Hz tones. The thin lines show the instantaneous amplitude waveform (snapshots at discrete time points in the stimulus cycle) at several time points, whereas the dotted line shows the basilar membrane displacement envelope over many time points. For each frequency, the traveling wave amplitude gradually increases from the base towards a maximum and then rapidly declines. The peak of the displacement envelope for the 8000 Hz tone is located near the base, the peak for 2000 Hz is located near the middle of the cochlea, and the peak for 200 Hz is located near the apex. The piano keyboard below the graph illustrates the tonotopic organization (frequency versus place) of the cochlea. The main difference between the piano keyboard and the traveling wave vibration pattern is that high level, low frequency sounds not only vibrate the apex of the cochlea but also the more basal region of the cochlea, albeit at a lower vibration amplitude.

The right ordinate of the 2000 Hz plot shows the phase lag at each point along the basilar membrane relative to the motion of the stapes. Here it can be seen that motion of the basilar membrane near the base is nearly in phase (0° phase lag) with the stapes; the phase lag of basilar membrane motion relative to the stapes increases with distance from the base of

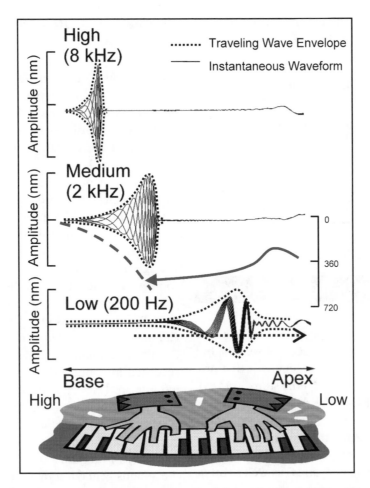

Figure 2–4. Schematics of traveling wave displacement along the basilar membrane (base to apex), for high frequency tones (8000 Hz), mid-frequency tones (2000 Hz), and low frequency tones (200 Hz). The dotted lines show the envelope of the basilar membrane response; note that the peak of the envelope is located near the base of the cochlea for high frequencies and near the apex for low frequencies. The thin lines show the instantaneous waveform of the traveling wave at different times. The piano keyboard below illustrates the tonotopic organization of the cochlea where high frequencies are coded near the base and low frequencies are coded near the apex. *Note.* Redrawn from "Anatomy and Physiology of the Peripheral Auditory System," by R. J.Salvi, W. Sun, and E. Lobarinas, 2007, in R. Roeser, H. Hosford-Dunn, and M. Valente (Eds.), *Audiology Diagnosis*, pp. 17–36, New York: Thieme. Used with permission.

the cochlea. Near the peak of the traveling wave envelope, basilar membrane motion lags behind stapes motion; in the example shown the phase lag is approx-imately 520°. Thus, the motion of apical regions of the cochlea lags behind more basal regions. The shift in the peak of the traveling wave envelope results in a frequency-to-place transformation or tonotopic organization.

KEY POINT

The cochlea acts like a spectrum analyzer that distributes the frequency components in a sound to different regions of the cochlea; the tonotopic organization of the auditory system is established in the cochlea.

OTOACOUSTIC EMISSIONS

Recent studies have shown that the inner ear not only receives sounds, but also acts as a sound a generator that produces otoacoustic emissions (OAEs). These OAEs are the result of "nonlinear" behavior in the inner ear. Nonlinear behavior means that given any two (or more) sounds (f_1 and f_2) in the input, the output will have f_1 and f_2 as well as other frequency components that were not in the original sound input. Tartini, the 18th century classical musician, exploited this phenomenon in his compositions (Jaramillo, Markin, & Hudspeth, 1993). The OHC electromotile response, driven by the voltage-sensitive motor protein, prestin, plus the +80 mV endolymphatic potential, is believed to be the source of OAEs in mammals. OAEs are generated in healthy ears but are reduced in amplitude or absent when the OHCs are damaged or the endolymphatic potential is reduced (Hofstetter, Ding, Powers, & Salvi, 1997; Siegel & Kim, 1982; Trautwein, Hofstetter, Wang, Salvi, & Nostrant, 1996). The most frequently investigated OAEs are described in the following sections.

Spontaneous Otoacoustic Emissions

Spontaneous otoacoustic emissions (SOAEs), as the name implies, occur spontaneously and can be recorded in the ear canal with a sensitive microphone connected to a narrowband spectrum analyzer. SOAEs typically occur as one or two narrowband acoustic signals. Figure 2–5a shows the SOAEs recorded from the ear canal of a chinchilla; the robust SOAEs recorded in this animal occurred near 4500 Hz. The 30 dB SPL SOAE was loud enough that it could be heard in a quiet room when the ear of the listener was placed near the animal's ear (Powers, Salvi, Wang, Spongr, & Qiu, 1995). SOAEs can only be recorded in a subpopulation of animals or humans. SOAEs can only be recorded in about 33% of normal hearing humans (Probst, Lonsbury-Martin, & Martin, 1991). It was once thought that SOAEs might represent the neuron-acoustic correlate of tinnitus; unfortunately, most individuals with SOAEs are unable to hear the sounds generated by their own ears (Glanville, Coles, & Sullivan, 1971). So far, SOAEs have been found to have little clinical value.

Distortion Product Otoacoustic Emissions

In the routine clinical assessment of distortion product otoacoustic emissions (DPOAE), two primary tones are presented to the ear through two miniature loudspeakers coupled to the ear canal along with a sensitive microphone that is used to record the primary tones as well any distortion sounds generated by the ear. The distortion generated in healthy

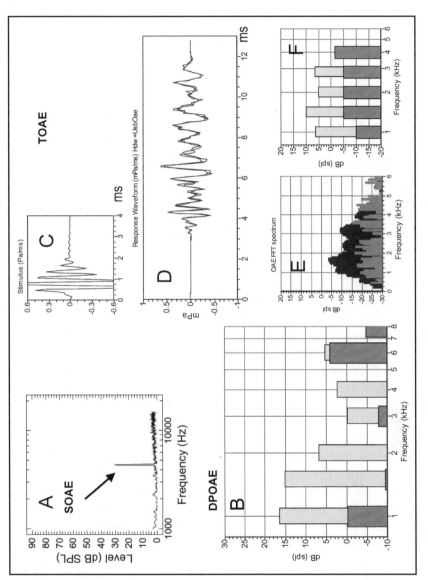

Figure 2–5. (A) Amplitude versus frequency spectrum recorded from the ear canal of a chinchilla using a sensitive microphone. (B) DPOAE amplitude (light gray) plotted as function of the geometric mean for f_1 and f_2 stimulus frequencies from 1000 Hz to 8000 Hz; dark gray bars show noise floor of the measurement system. (C) Pressure versus time waveform of click stimulus used to elicit the TOAE. (D) TOAE pressure versus time waveform obtained with the click stimulus shown in panel C. (E) Spectral analysis showing the sound pressure level (dB SPL) versus frequency. Dark area shows spectrum of TOAEs; gray areas show spectrum of the background noise of the measurement system and subject. (F) Bar graph showing the sound pressure level in narrow bands of noise located at frequencies between 1000 Hz and 4000 Hz.

human ears is typically elicited by two primary tones, f_1 and f_2, where f_1 is the lower frequency and f_2 the higher frequency. The optimal conditions for eliciting DPOAEs are with an f_2/f_1 ratio of approximately 1.2 and when the intensity (L1) of f_1 is approximately +10 dB greater than the intensity (L2) of f_2. When f_1 and f_2 are presented to a normal ear with intact OHCs, the microphone not only picks up the primary tones, f_1 and f_2, but also intermodulation distortion tones, the largest of which occur at frequencies $2f_1-f_2$. For example, if primary tones of 2000 Hz and 2400 Hz are presented to the ear, the $2f_1-f_2$ distortion product occurs at 1600 Hz. In some cases, the intensity of $2f_1-f_2$ is only 30 to 40 dB below the level of the primary tones.

Figure 2–5b shows the amplitude of $2f_1-f_2$ DPOAEs that were measured in a 35-year-old adult male when the f_2/f_1 ratio was 1.22 and L1 was 75 dB and L2 was 70 dB. DPOAE amplitude was plotted as the geometric mean frequency of f_1 and f_2 from 1000 to 8000 Hz. DPOAE amplitude decreased from about 15 dB SPL at 1000 Hz to 0 dB SPL at 3000 Hz; the amplitude increased to 5 dB SPL at 6000 Hz and then disappeared below the noise floor of the measuring system (dark gray) at higher frequencies. The absence of any DPOAEs above 6000 Hz suggests that most of the OHCs are damaged or missing at the high frequencies in this individual. A plot of DPOAE amplitude as function of f_2/f_1 frequency is often referred to as a DPgram because of similarities to the audiogram. In addition to a DPgram, the DPOAE input/output function can be measured at a specific f_2/f_1 ratio by varying the intensity of L1 and L2 from low to high. DPOAE amplitude increases at low-to-moderate intensities but saturates at higher levels (Eddins, Zuskov, & Salvi, 1999; Probst et al., 1991).

Transient Otoacoustic Emissions

Transient otoacoustic emissions (TOAEs) are elicited with transient signals such as the click shown in Figure 2–5c, which has a duration of approximately 2 ms (Kemp, 1978). When the click stimulus enters the cochlea, the spectral component of the click is distributed spatially and temporally (high frequencies arrive at the base first, low frequencies arrive at the apex later) along the length of the cochlea. The high frequency components in the click activate OHCs in the base of the cochlea first; the OHCs generate high frequency TOAEs that propagate in the reverse direction back to the ear canal. The mid-frequency components in the click activate the OHCs in the middle of the cochlea; the OHCs in the middle of the cochlea generate mid-frequency TOAEs that propagate back to the ear canal a little while after the high frequency TOAEs. The low frequency TOAEs emerge even later than the high frequencies. Figure 2–5d shows the temporal dispersion of the click-evoked TOAEs. The high-frequency component emerges around 4 ms, whereas the low frequencies emerge around 12 ms following the onset of the acoustic click. Note that the time between peaks is shorter at the beginning of the waveform than at the end, and this is consistent with the emergence of high frequencies first and low frequencies later.

The spectral content of the click-evoked TOAEs shown in Figure 2–5d can be analyzed by performing a Fourier analysis of the waveform; this analysis gives the raw TOAEs shown in Figure 2–5e. The dark band in Figure 2–5e shows the spectrum of the TOAEs and the shaded portion shows the noise level of the measurement system. The lightly shaded bars in Figure 2–5f show the SPL in half octave bands of the TOAEs from 1000 Hz to 6000 Hz; the dark bars show the noise floor of the measuring system. The amplitude of the TOAEs ranges from 5 to 10 dB from 1000 to 3000 Hz and is well above the noise floor; however, the TOAEs are absent above 3000 Hz. This suggests that OHCs are functional at 3000 Hz and below, but the lack of TOAEs above 3000 Hz suggest that OHCs are damaged in the high frequency region of the cochlea.

When the TOAEs were first discovered, they were referred to as cochlear echoes because of the time delay between the original acoustic signal (Figure 2–5c) and the TOAEs that first appeared around 4 ms continuing on to 12 ms. Unfortunately, this terminology gives the mistaken impression that the TOAEs are a passive reflection of sound from the cochlea. However, the TOAEs cannot be an echo because (a) the amplitude of the TOAEs increases nonlinearly with increasing intensity and (b) the TOAEs disappear when the cochlea is damaged by metabolic inhibitors, acoustic trauma, or ototoxic drugs (Kemp, 1978).

KEY POINT

DPOAEs and TOAEs can be used clinically to evaluate the functional status of the OHCs. When the OHCs are damaged or the endolymphatic potential is reduced, DPOAE and TOAE amplitudes are greatly reduced.

AUDITORY NERVE FIBER RESPONSES

The VIII cranial nerve is referred to as the auditory nerve and it is the route by which neurological impulses get from the cochlea to the auditory cortex in the brain. By using extremely fine microelectrodes, it is possible to record the activity from single auditory nerve fibers that transmit information from the hair cells to the cochlear nucleus (see Figure 2–1d). When a microelectrode is inserted into the auditory nerve, it is possible to record the all-or-none spike discharges from individual nerve fibers (Figure 2–6a). Most auditory nerve fibers discharge spontaneously in the absence of sound; individual auditory nerve fibers discharge spontaneously at rates that vary from nearly 0 spikes per second to as high as 125 spikes per second. Figure 2–6b is a schematic histogram showing the proportion of neurons with various spontaneous rates. The distribution is bimodal. A large percentage have either very low spontaneous rates (<1 spike/s) or very high spontaneous rates (>18 spikes/s), whereas only a small percentage have rates between 1 and 18 spikes/s (Salvi, Perry, Hamernik, & Henderson, 1982). Spontaneous activity is believed to arise from the spontaneous release of neurotransmitter, most likely glutamate, from the IHCs onto the afferent dendrite of an auditory nerve fiber.

Because most auditory nerve fibers (~90%) make one-to-one synaptic contact with a single IHC (Spoendlin, 1972), the neural response of each fiber reflects the neural output from a discrete region along the cochlear partition. The output of each fiber can be "interrogated" by presenting tone bursts at different frequencies and intensities to determine which frequency-intensity combinations are just capable of activating it, that is, the frequency-threshold tuning curve. Figure 2–6c is a schematic showing the lowest intensity of the tone burst needed to activate the fiber at different frequencies.

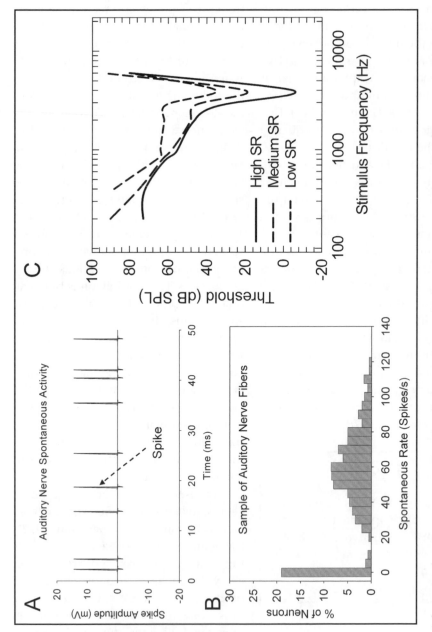

Figure 2–6. **(A)** Schematic showing spontaneous spike discharges from a single auditory nerve fiber. **(B)** Schematic showing the proportion of auditory nerve fibers with different spontaneous discharge rates. **(C)** Schematic showing representative frequency-threshold tuning curves from auditory nerve fibers with high, medium, or low spontaneous rates. Tuning curves are shown for neurons with characteristic frequency (CF) near 4000 Hz. High spontaneous rate units have the lowest thresholds and low spontaneous rate units have the highest thresholds. *Note.* From "Anatomy and Physiology of the Peripheral Auditory System," by R. J. Salvi, W. Sun, and E. Lobarinas, 2007, in R. Roeser, H. Hosford-Dunn, and M. Valente (Eds.), *Audiology Diagnosis*, pp. 17–36, New York: Thieme. Used with permission.

Results are shown for 3 units, one with a low, another with a medium, and a third with a high spontaneous rate. The unit with a high spontaneous rate has a frequency-threshold tuning curve with a sharply tuned low threshold tip near 4000 Hz; the lowest threshold in the tip is referred to as the characteristic frequency (CF). The sound intensity needed to produce a threshold response increases rapidly as the frequency moves above. As the frequency moves below CF, the sound intensity needed to elicit a response initially increases rapidly; however, the increase in threshold becomes more gradual one to two octaves below CF, resulting in a more broadly tuned, low frequency tail. Thus, the typical auditory nerve fiber has a low threshold, narrowly tuned tip flanked by a steeply rising slope on the high frequency side of CF. The slope below CF initially rises steeply, but then flattens out to form a high threshold, broadly tuned tail. The frequency-threshold tuning curves for low, medium, and high spontaneous rate neurons have a similar shape; however, the threshold at a particular CF can vary by as much as 60 dB for different fibers. Neurons with high spontaneous rates have the lowest thresholds, whereas those with the lowest spontaneous rates have the highest thresholds (Salvi et al., 1982).

KEY POINT

The tuning curve of each auditory nerve fiber is focused on a narrow range of frequencies. However, humans can hear over a wide range of frequencies because some fibers are tuned to low frequencies and others to mid- or high frequencies, which spans the entire range of hearing.

After recording from a fiber, a dye can be injected into the neuron to the location and type of hair cell it innervates. These studies have revealed two important facts. First, the CF of the labeled neuron was correlated with the position along the length of the cochlea. High CF neurons innervated hair cells in the base of the cochlea, whereas low CF fibers innervated hair cells in the apex of the cochlea consistent with the traveling wave (see Figure 2–4). These results indicate that the tonotopic arrangement of the cochlea is maintained by auditory nerve fibers as they pass from the cochlea into the cochlear nucleus. Second, all dye labeled fibers that responded to sound were traced back to IHCs; none were found to contact OHCs (Liberman, 1982; Robertson, 1984). These results suggest that virtually all of the acoustic information transmitted to the central auditory system are conveyed by the type I auditory nerve fibers. Apparently, type II fibers that contact OHCs have not been shown to produce spike discharges in response to sound (Robertson, 1984).

When a tone burst is presented within the boundaries of the fibers' response region, the fiber will produce spike discharges over the duration of the stimulus. The discharge pattern over time can be mapped out by counting the number of spikes that occur at different time points before, during, and following the stimulus. The spike counts are plotted as a function of time from stimulus onset to construct a poststimulus time histogram. Figure 2–7a shows a series of poststimulus time histograms obtained with a 200 ms tone burst presented at sound intensity below, near, and well above threshold. At 18 dB SPL, the neuron's spike rate during the stimulus is nearly the same as that following the stimulus, indicating that the

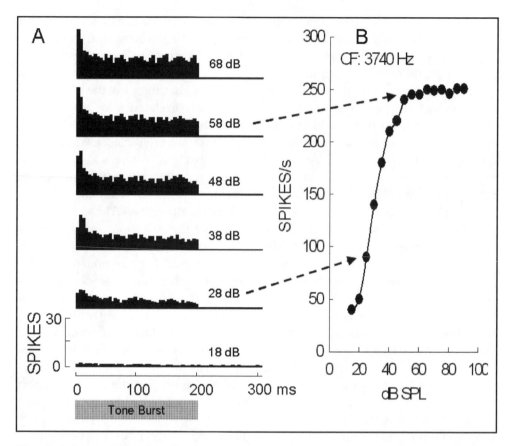

Figure 2–7. (**A**) Schematic showing representative poststimulus time histogram (PSTH) of spike count versus time from an auditory nerve fiber stimulated with a 200 ms duration tone burst. Sound intensity increased from 18 to 68 dB SPL in 10 dB steps. (**B**) Schematic showing spike rate (spikes/s) versus stimulus level. Spike rate increases rapidly from 23 to 58 dB SPL and then plateaus at higher stimulus levels. *Note.* From "Anatomy and Physiology of the Peripheral Auditory System," by R. J. Salvi , W. Sun, and E. Lobarinas, 2007, in R. Roeser, H. Hosford-Dunn, and M. Valente (Eds.), *Audiology Diagnosis*, pp. 17–36, New York: Thieme. Used with permission.

firing rate is below or near threshold. When the intensity increases to 28 dB SPL, the firing rate at stimulus onset increases and then gradually declines over the next 25 ms to a steady state level that continues over the duration of the stimulus. When the stimulus is turned off, the spike rate rapidly declines to its spontaneous rate. Further increases in intensity cause the onset firing rate and steady state firing rate to increase (see Figure 2-7a).

The decrease in firing rate from the peak to the plateau region is believed to reflect neural adaptation caused by depletion of the pool of available neurotransmitter vesicles released from the hair cells onto the type I afferent dendrites. When the stimulus is turned off, the vesicular pool is replenished, allowing the auditory nerve fiber to again respond robustly at stimulus onset. The dynamic range refers to the range of sound intensities over which the spike rate increases as the intensity increases. The dynamic range for the neuron shown in Figure 2–7b is approximately 40 dB. The dynamic range of most auditory nerve fibers ranges from 30 to 50 dB. This means that a single fiber can unambiguously encode changes in sound intensity only over a 30 to 50 dB range, far less than that dynamic range of loudness that spans approximately 130 dB. However, because the distribution of thresholds at a particular CF varies by as much as 60 dB, low threshold, high spontaneous rate fibers could code for loudness changes at low-to-moderate intensities, whereas high threshold, low spontaneous rate fibers could code for loudness at high intensities. Thus, the dynamic range of an individual neuron combined with the 60 dB range of thresholds at CF provides for a method of coding loudness over a range of 110–130 dB.

CENTRAL AUDITORY PATHWAY

The output of the auditory nerve is relayed to neurons in the cochlear nuclei (see Figure 2–1d). The inputs to the cochlear nuclei are mainly from the same side, or unilateral. The output from the cochlear nuclei is relayed on to the superior olivary complex on the same side as well as the opposite side of the brainstem. The relative intensity and time of arrival of signals coming into the superior olivary complex from the two ears are used to compute the location of sounds in space, or sound localization. Sounds emitted from a loudspeaker located on the right side of the head will arrive at the right ear first and the left ear approximately 800 μs later. Neurons in the superior olivary complex and higher levels of the auditory pathway can detect these time differences and use the information to compute the location of the sound source. Interaural time differences play an important role in determining the location of a sound source at frequencies below 2000 Hz.

Sounds emitted from a loudspeaker located on the right side of the head must pass around the head to reach the opposite ear. Long wavelength, low frequency sounds wrap around the head to reach the opposite ear; consequently, the interaural difference between the two ears is relatively small at low frequencies. However, as frequencies increase and the wavelength of sound becomes shorter, the head tends to block the transmission of sound to the opposite ear, creating a head shadow effect. At high frequencies, the interaural difference in sound intensity can be as high as 20 dB near 10,000 Hz. Neurons in the superior olivary complex and higher parts of the auditory pathway can compute the interaural intensity differences at high frequencies in order to determine the location of a sound source.

The output of the superior olive is relayed to the lateral lemniscus and then to the inferior colliculus, another important binaural processing center that is located in the midbrain. The output of the inferior colliculus is relayed to the medial geniculate body located at the back of the thalamus and then to the auditory cortex, which is involved in recognizing and interpreting complex sounds such as speech and music.

Acknowledgments. This research was supported in part by grants from the National Institutes of Health (R01 DC00630 and R01 DC009091).

REFERENCES

Ades, H. W., & Engstrom, H. (1974). Anatomy of the inner ear. In W. D. Keidel & W. D. Neff (Eds.), *Handbook of sensory physiology* (Vol. V[I], pp. 125-128). New York: Springer Verlag.

Bekesy, G. (1960). *Experiments in hearing.* New York: John Wiley & Sons.

Bosher, S. K., & Warren, R. L. (1968). Observations on the electrochemistry of the cochlear endolymph of the rat: A quantitative study of its electrical potential and ionic composition as determined by means of flame spectrophotometry. *Proceedings of the Royal Society of London, Series B Biological Sciences, 171*(23), 227-247.

Dallos, P., Billone, M. C., Durrant, J. D., Wang, C. Y., & Raynor, S. (1972). Cochlear inner and outer hair cells: Functional differences. *Science, 177,* 356-358.

Dallos, P., & Fakler, B. (2002). Prestin, a new type of motor protein. *Nature Reviews Molecular Cell Biology, 3*(2), 104-111.

Durrant, J. D., Wang, J., Ding, D. L., & Salvi, R. J. (1998). Are inner or outer hair cells the source of summating potentials recorded from the round window? *Journal of the Acoustical Society of America, 104*(1), 370-377.

Eddins, A. C., Zuskov, M., & Salvi, R. J. (1999). Changes in distortion product otoacoustic emissions during prolonged noise exposure. *Hearing Research, 127*(1-2), 119-128.

Gale, J. E., & Ashmore, J. F. (1997). An intrinsic frequency limit to the cochlear amplifier. *Nature, 389*(6646), 63-66.

Glanville, J. D., Coles, R. R. A., & Sullivan, B. M. (1971). A family with high-tonal objective tinnitus. *Journal of Otolaryngology, 85,* 1-10.

Hofstetter, P., Ding, D., Powers, N., & Salvi, R. J. (1997). Quantitative relationship of carboplatin dose to magnitude of inner and outer hair cell loss and the reduction in distortion product otoacoustic emission

amplitude in chinchillas. *Hearing Research, 112*(1-2), 199-215.

Holley, M. C., & Ashmore, J. F. (1988). A cytoskeletal spring in cochlear outer hair cells. *Nature, 335*(6191), 635-637.

Hood, L. J. (1990). Update on frequency specificity of AEP measurements. *Journal of the American Academy of Audiology, 1*(3), 125-129.

Hudspeth, A. J. (1992). Hair-bundle mechanics and a model for mechanoelectrical transduction by hair cells. *Society of General Physiologists Series, 47,* 357-370.

Jaramillo, F., Markin, V. S., & Hudspeth, A. J. (1993). Auditory illusions and the single hair cell. *Nature, 364*(6437), 527-529.

Kemp, D. (1978). Stimulated acoustic emissions from within the human auditory system. *Journal of the Acoustical Society of America, 64,* 1386-1391.

Khanna, S. M., & Leonard, D. G. B. (1982). Basilar membrane tuning in the cat cochlea. *Science, 215,* 305-306.

Liberman, M. C. (1982). Single-neuron labeling in the cat auditory nerve. *Science, 216,* 1239-1241.

Liberman, M. C., Gao, J., He, D. Z., Wu, X., Jia, S., & Zuo, J. (2002). Prestin is required for electromotility of the outer hair cell and for the cochlear amplifier. *Nature, 419*(6904), 300-304.

Nedzelnitsky, V. (1980). Sound pressures in the basal turn of the cat cochlea. *Journal of the Acoustical Society of America, 68*(6), 1676-1689.

Nuttall, A. L., Dolan, D. F., & Avinash, G. (1991). Laser Doppler velocimetry of basilar membrane vibration. *Hearing Research, 51*(2), 203-213.

Powers, N. L., Salvi, R. J., Wang, J., Spongr, V., & Qiu, C. X. (1995). Elevation of auditory thresholds by spontaneous cochlear oscillations. *Nature, 375*(6532), 585-587.

Probst, R., Lonsbury-Martin, B. L., & Martin, G. K. (1991). A review of otoacoustic emissions. *Journal of the Acoustical Society of America, 89,* 2027-2067.

Robertson, D. (1984). Horseradish peroxidase injection of physiologically characterized afferent and efferent neurons in the guinea pig spiral ganglion. *Hearing Research, 15,* 113–121.

Ryan, A., & Dallos, P. (1975). Effect of absence of cochlear outer hair cells on behavioural auditory threshold. *Nature, 253*(5486), 44–46.

Salvi, R. J., Perry, J., Hamernik, R. P., & Henderson, D. (Eds.). (1982). *Relationship between cochlear pathologies and auditory nerve and behavioral responses following acoustic trauma.* New York: Raven Press.

Sellick, P. M., Patuzzi, R., & Johnstone, B. M. (1982). Measurement of basilar membrane motion in the guinea pig using the Mossbauer technique. *Journal of the Acoustical Society of America, 72*(1), 131–141.

Shaw, E. A. G. (1974). Transformation of sound pressure level from the free field to the eardrum in the horizontal plane. *Journal of the Acoustical Society of America, 56*(6), 1848–1861.

Shaw, N. A. (1995). The temporal relationship between the brainstem and primary cortical auditory evoked potentials. *Progress in Neurobiology, 47*(2), 95–103.

Siegel, J. H., & Kim, D. O. (1982). Cochlear biomechanics: Vulnerability to acoustic trauma and other alterations as seen in neural responses and ear-canal sound pressure. In R. P. Hamernik, D. Henderson, & R. J. Salvi (Eds.), *New perspectives on noise-induced hearing loss* (pp. 137–151). New York: Raven Press.

Spoendlin, H. (1972). Innervation densities of the cochlea. *Acta Oto-Laryngololica, 67,* 235–248.

Starr, A., Picton, T. W., Sininger, Y., Hood, L. J., & Berlin, C. I. (1996). Auditory neuropathy. *Brain, 119*(Pt. 3), 741–753.

Trautwein, P., Hofstetter, P., Wang, J., Salvi, R., & Nostrant, A. (1996). Selective inner hair cell loss does not alter distortion product otoacoustic emissions. *Hearing Research, 96*(1-2), 71–82.

Wang, J., Powers, N. L., Hofstetter, P., Trautwein, P., Ding, D., & Salvi, R. (1997). Effects of selective inner hair cell loss on auditory nerve fiber threshold, tuning and spontaneous and driven discharge rate. *Hearing Research, 107*(1-2), 67–82.

3 The Medical Aspects of Otologic Damage from Noise in Musicians

BY KENNETH EINHORN

Every day in the United States, an otolaryngologist encounters a patient with hearing loss that is caused in part or in whole by loud noise exposure. Approximately 10 million Americans suffer from hearing loss attributed to damage from excessive noise exposure (National Institutes of Health [NIH], 1990). The physician is also familiar with some (but maybe not all) of the other adverse medical conditions that can arise from this type of damage. Disorders arising from noise induced otologic damage (NIOD) include auditory disturbances and, potentially, vestibular dysfunction (Table 3-1).

For the patient who has worked in an industrial setting associated with excessive noise levels, the source of the damage seems obvious to the otolaryngologist. However, many otolaryngologists (and other physicians) may not be aware that these medical conditions exist and are of particular concern in the performing arts, especially for musicians.

In one recent study (Kahari, Zachau, Eklof, Sandsjo, & Moller, 2003), manifestations of one or more of these disorders were found in 74% of the 139 rock/jazz musicians studied. The implications of

Table 3–1. Disorders Arising from Noise Induced Otologic Damage

Auditory Disturbances
  Noise Induced Hearing Loss
  Tinnitus
  Hyperacusis
  Diplacusis
  Recruitment

Vestibular Dysfunction
  Vertigo
  Disequilibrium

NIOD are important for all of us, but they are of particular importance to musicians. Musicians' hearing necessities, as related to their livelihoods, are much greater than those of other professions, and their hearing-related injuries can become severe or possibly career-ending disabilities (Sataloff, 1991).

This chapter will provide hearing health care professionals with the understanding of (a) the medical disorders arising from NIOD as they relate to the musician, (b) the musician-specific aspects of the medical and audiologic evaluation, treatment options, and counseling of a musician with noise related damage, and (c) the need for and means of prevention available to musicians.

KEY POINT

Otologic damage from chronic loud noise (including music) exposure can lead to disorders of auditory disturbances (noise induced hearing loss, tinnitus, hyperacusis, diplacusis, and recruitment) and vestibular dysfunction.

NIOD DISORDERS

Music Induced Hearing Loss

Gradual hearing loss resulting from chronic loud noise exposure is termed *noise induced hearing loss* (NIHL). When the gradual hearing loss is a result of chronic exposure to loud music, it is termed *music induced hearing loss* (MIHL). For a full discussion of the biomechanics and the biochemistry of NIHL, the reader is referred to Chapter 2.

As indicated through a review of the medical and audiologic literature, MIHL occurs among musicians with varying incidences depending on the type of music played (i.e., classical, rock, or jazz). Incidences of hearing loss reported among classical musicians range from 4% to 58% with most of the losses being mild (Axelsson & Lindgren, 1981; Chesky & Henoch, 2000; Karlsson, Lundquist, & Olaussen, 1983; Ostri, Eller, Dahlin, & Skylv, 1989; Westmore & Eversden, 1981). Incidences of hearing loss reported among rock and pop musicians range from 13%

to 30% (Axelsson & Lindgren, 1978; Chesky & Henoch, 2000; Hart, Geltman, Schupbach, & Santucci, 1987). Dey (1970) reported severe temporary threshold shifts in listeners exposed to rock music at 110 dBA and, based on damage risk criterion, "16% would be adversely and probably permanently affected" (p. 469). This raises the specter that loud rock music may lead to more severe losses than the mild ones noted for classical musicians.

The literature is quite clear that sound pressure levels that musicians routinely face lie within potentially hazardous ranges, extending up to 120 to 130 dBA only 3 feet from the speaker in amplified rock/pop bands (Hart et al., 1987), 83 to 112 dBA on stage in various orchestras (Sataloff, 1991), and 80 to 101 dBA on stage in jazz, blues, and country and western bands (Chasin, 1996). Furthermore, for rock/jazz/pop music performances, there is not much variation in the sound levels during the performance as compared to classical music (Hart et al., 1987). Therefore, on the average, rock music is louder than classical music because there are not as many quiet passages in the arrangements (Gunderson, Moline, & Catalano, 1997).

Most musicians practice or perform up to 8 or more hours a day, depending on how close they are to the day or week of performance. Also, they enjoy listening to the music of others. These factors in addition to the sound levels they encounter, as noted above, suggest a strong causal relationship between their chronic loud music exposure and their NIHL.

One of the most common problems that people with NIHL experience is difficulty in speech comprehension, especially in the presence of background noise. This, of course, is secondary to hearing loss in the high frequencies. However, high frequency hearing loss is particularly detrimental for musicians and singers because they must also accurately match frequencies over a broad range, including frequencies above those required for speech comprehension. It may lead to excessively loud playing at higher pitches and, thus, to an unacceptable performance. It can also lead to arm and wrist strain, as in the example of the violinist who, in order to compensate for his hearing loss, may bow harder or "overbow" (Chasin, 1996). Furthermore, the loss of color and clarity, especially in the higher tones, can impair one's ability to enjoy listening to music.

KEY POINT

These disorders exist among musicians with varying incidences and can potentially represent debilitating or career-ending injuries.

Unlike NIHL that is seen in the industrial setting, MIHL in musicians is often asymmetric—probably relating to the position of their own instrument (or others' instruments) and/or the position of onstage monitors or amplifiers to their ears. For instance, in the rock drummer, it tends to be worse in the left ear owing to its closer proximity to the high hat cymbals. It also tends to be worse in the left ear of violinists and worse in the right ear of flute and piccolo players. Because of this imbalance, it is not unusual for these musicians to complain of distortion even in their better ear (Chasin, 1996).

Tinnitus

Tinnitus is the perception of sound in the ear when no external source exists. It is the most common condition accompanying NIHL. According to the American Tinnitus Association, up to 90% of all tinnitus patients have some degree of NIHL. Tinnitus is usually (but not always) high pitched, nonpulsatile, and subjective (perceived only by the sufferer). It commonly precedes subjective awareness of hearing loss.

Tinnitus can get so loud that it can be more debilitating than the hearing loss itself. Numerous rock musicians have admitted to suffering from tinnitus to the point that they have limited their live performances or retired from the music industry altogether. Laitinen (2005) found tinnitus in 37% of classical musicians within a study group consisting of five major orchestras. Tinnitus is particularly damaging to the players of string instruments, especially higher pitched instruments like violins and violas. It also seems that continued exposure to music at any volume level can intensify its loudness and intolerability.

Hyperacusis

Hyperacusis is the term used to describe a painful hypersensitivity or decreased tolerance to normal sound. Between 25% and 40% of patients with hyperacusis also experience tinnitus (Shiley, Folmer, & McMenomey, 2005). Hyperacusis can lead to phonophobia, a fear of sound regardless of its volume. As a result, much of the day can be spent monitoring sound levels in one's immediate surroundings or overprotecting one's ears by the daily overuse of earplugs or earmuffs from everyday sounds. This can then lead to further hypersensitization. A vicious cycle of overprotection, hyperacusis, and phonophobia can then develop (Shiley et al., 2005).

Laitinen (2005) also noted that 43% of the classical musicians in his study were found to have hyperacusis. The potential devastating and/or career-ending consequences for a musician noted with tinnitus hold true for hyperacusis as well. Furthermore, the association of hyperacusis and phonophobia can lead to the musician's overuse and improper selection of hearing protection, thus complicating his ability to perform and leading to an impaired performance.

Diplacusis and Recruitment

Diplacusis is the abnormal perception of sound, either in pitch or in time, so that one sound is heard as two. It can also refer to the phenomenon where an increase in a frequency of a particular sound is perceived only as an increase in loudness; the pitch seems to stay the same. Diplacusis may cause a musical note to sound flat or cause a musician to play out of tune (Chasin, 1996). Recruitment is when there is a sharp increase in a sound's perceived loudness associated with only a relatively small increase in the sound's actual intensity. As a result, even mildly loud sounds from the musician's instrument may cause him to perceive it as painfully loud (Chasin, 1996). It is also of interest to note that the presence of diplacusis and recruitment is quite common in Ménière's disease.

Vestibular Dysfunction

Because it shares a membranous labyrinth, similar hair cell microstructure, and a common arterial supply with the auditory system, the vestibular apparatus is at risk for damage from loud noise

exposure (Lonsbury-Martin & Martin, 2005). While this remains a controversial topic, several studies over the past 20 years support the association of loud noise and vestibular disturbance including disequilibrium and abnormal vestibular function tests (Shupak et al., 1994; J. Ylikoski, Juntunen, Matikainen, M. Ylikoski, & Ojala, 1988). Golz et al. (2001) found clinical evidence of vestibular damage among 258 military subjects exposed to intense noise only when there was asymmetric hearing loss present. This is of particular concern for musicians as MIHL is often asymmetric.

MEDICAL HISTORY

In obtaining a medical history from the musician, the otolaryngologist must determine if any of the disorders discussed are present and, if so, the date of onset, type of onset, subsequent progression, and the presence of other otologic symptoms (otalgia, aural fullness, and otorrhea). In those patients presenting with tinnitus, an inquiry is made as to whether the tinnitus is intermittent versus continuous, or pulsatile versus nonpulsatile. Pulsatile or noncontinuous tinnitus commonly arises from a vascular source or abnormality.

The physician must ask about factors that can contribute to or predispose to NIHL (Table 3–2). While the data on some of these factors are inconclusive, others have been well documented and deserve special mention. Smokers are at higher risk of developing NIHL, most likely from cardiovascular damage as a result of smoking. Noise in conjunction with ototoxic medications produces greater damage than each stimulus applied separately (Lonsbury-Martin & Martin, 2005). Aspi-

Table 3–2. Factors that Contribute or Predispose to NIHL

Age

Chemical Agents
  Environmental
  Industrial

Diabetes Mellitus

Genetic Factors
  Genetic Susceptibility
  Gender

Hyperlipoproteinemia

Ototoxic Medications

Presbycusis

Recreational Noise
  Shooting
  Power Tools
  Motor Sports
  Listening to Loud Music
  Arcade Games

Risk Factors for Cardiovascular Disease

Smoking

(i.e., Ménière's disease, perilymphatic fistula, otosclerosis) should be sought. Also, the otolaryngologist should ask about nonotologic diseases known to cause other types of hearing loss (i.e., stroke, head trauma, cardiovascular disease, syphilis, retrocochlear neoplasm, severe hypothyroidism, and autoimmune disorders) as well as tinnitus and hyperacusis (temporomandibular joint syndrome, migraine, Lyme disease, Bell's palsy, vascular abnormalities, and depression).

KEY POINT

In the medical examination and testing of a musician with one or more of these disorders, the examining otolaryngologist must be aware of the musician-specific aspects to the medical history taking, physical examination, and auditory assessment.

An inquiry into one's noise exposure must be included. For a musician, not only does it include the number of years playing, but also the typical practice and performance schedule history, position of instrument, and position in relation to the other musicians or amplifiers/speakers/monitors. A discussion should pursue the nonoccupational music exposure, especially live performances and personal MP3 or CD player usage.

rin, non steroidal anti-inflammatories, and "loop" diuretics cause reversible hearing loss and tinnitus. However, aminoglycoside antibiotics and platinum derivative antineoplastic medications lead to permanent damage. Some studies have shown similar synergistic damaging effects of noise and such environmental pollutants as carbon monoxide and hydrogen cyanide (Fechter, Chen, & Rao, 2002) as well as certain industrial chemicals including organic solvents, metals, and certain noxious gases (Morata & Little, 2002).

As part of the review of past medical history, any history of otologic diseases

PHYSICAL EXAMINATION

A general head and neck physical examination is performed with special attention to the otologic exam. Pneumatic otoscopy, tuning forks, and microscopic visualization should be included. An otoneurologic examination for objective tinnitus, gait, balance, and vertigo may be needed if symptoms indicate. It may be necessary to order an MRI if retro-cochlear neoplasm/pathology is suspected. A CT scan may be needed if temporal bone pathology is suspected. Disease-specific blood tests should be obtained if there is suspicion for any of the previously noted diseases.

AUDIOLOGIC ASSESSMENT

Conventional audiometric testing is obtained. Particular attention is directed to the audiogram, looking for the presence of a sensorineural hearing loss within the 3000 Hz to 6000 Hz region but, for a musician, not necessarily a 4000 Hz notch (typical for industrial NIHL). As previously noted and as discussed in Chapter 1, asymmetry of this high frequency loss is not an uncommon finding in musicians.

Of course, once a hearing loss is detected on the audiogram, cochlear damage has been established. With the advent and widespread availability of otoacoustic emissions (OAE) testing, we now have a means of early identification and possible prevention of MIHL (Hall & Bulla, 1999). OAEs are sounds that are measured in the external auditory canal and produced by the active motility of outer hair cells (OHCs) in response to a stimulus. They are extremely sensitive to even the most subtle changes in function of the OHCs, which are primarily involved in the beginning stages of NIHL, and can indicate cochlear dysfunction before clinically significant damage develops (Lonsbury-Martin & Martin, 2005).

Lastly, if vertigo or disequilibrium is present, vestibular function tests are obtained.

TREATMENT

Treatment of NIHL/MIHL

Currently there are no FDA approved medications to treat or prevent NIHL. However, advances in the preclinical, animal-based experimental investigations of certain compounds have led to the belief that medications with otoprotective capability against noise may be available in the not-so-distant future. The interest in most of these compounds is based on the popular hypothesis that the mechanism of injury in NIHL is cellular metabolic exhaustion with associated release of damaging free radicals and oxidants. While a full discussion of the various compounds being studied is beyond the scope of this chapter, most agents fall into the category of antioxidants (e.g., glutathione, N-acetyl-cysteine), antioxidant enzymes (ebselen), mitochondrial stabilizers (such as acetyl-L-carnitine), or glutamate antagonists (carbamathione) (Lynch & Kil, 2005). Until these agents pass through successful human clinical trials and become readily available, the treatment for MIHL among musicians remains rehabilitative, employing the use of hearing instruments.

Therefore, it is of utmost importance that the otolaryngologist discusses means of prevention with the musician. The use of high fidelity hearing protection devices should be recommended, including recommendations for specific types according to specific instruments and/or musical venue. Environmental modifications to reduce music exposure should be included in the discussion when appropriate. (The reader is referred to a full discussion of these two aspects found elsewhere in this book.) Additionally, all musicians should be advised to refrain from unprotected, nonoccupational loud noise exposure and to carefully monitor their recreational music exposure. Ototoxic medication should be avoided. Also, as part of prevention measures, medical disorders that contribute or predispose to NIHL (as discussed) should be medically treated.

KEY POINT

While preclinical investigations of certain compounds do seem to indicate that otoprotective medications may be on the near horizon, currently there is no medical cure for music induced hearing loss in the musician. Rehabilitative treatment utilizing hearing instruments remains the mainstay of therapy.

Treatment of Tinnitus

What determines whether treatment for tinnitus in musicians is indicated is the severity of the condition. Tinnitus severity can be quantified in many ways, the most utilized of which are the Tinnitus Handicap Inventory and the Tinnitus Severity Index (Seidman & Jacobson, 1996). Current treatment options for tinnitus are summarized in Table 3–3. Some patients require a multimodality strategy approach for optimal management.

Currently there is no drug that has been shown to cure tinnitus. However, many studies indicate that certain medications can reduce the tinnitus severity for some patients. The most common medications used are amitriptyline (Elavil), alprazolam (Xanax), diazepam (Valium), and histamine (Seidman & Jacobson, 1996). All of these medications possess side effects (e.g., sedation, dry mouth, etc.) that may impair a musician's per-

Table 3–3. Treatment Options for Tinnitus

Amplification (Hearing Aids)

Biofeedback

Counseling

Drug Therapy
    Antidepressants
    Antianxiety agents
    Antihistamines
    Anticonvulsants
    Anesthetics

Electrical Stimulation

Homeopathic Therapy
    Niacin
    Histamine
    Ginkgo Biloba
    Vitamin B
    Magnesium or Zinc
    Acupuncture

Masking Techniques
    In-the-Ear Sound Generators
    Sound Pillows
    CD/Radio

Tinnitus Retraining Therapy (TRT)

Temporomandibular Joint Treatment

formance and, therefore, must be discussed with the musician before prescribing and monitored.

The treatment option that seems to be the most popular among tinnitus centers in the United States and Europe is Tinnitus Retraining Therapy (TRT). Developed and described by Drs. Jastreboff and Hazell, it is an outgrowth of the neurophysiologic theory of tinnitus. TRT uses a combination of counseling and low level, broadband sound generators to achieve the habituation (to become unaware) of tinnitus (Jastreboff, Gray, & Gold, 1996). Jastreboff has treated over 800 patients and reports a success rate of 82% (Jastreboff & Jastreboff, 2003), a result that has been substantiated by various reports worldwide.

Treatment of Hyperacusis

Treatment options for hyperacusis remain limited. TRT is the most successful means of treating hyperacusis with 80 to 90% of patients reporting marked improvement (Jastreboff & Jastreboff, 2003). An alternative method is desensitization utilizing low frequency sound, or pink sound, delivered either through special fitted sound generators or on a compact disc.

Patients need to be counseled to be weaned off wearing earplugs or ear muffs in environments where they are not needed, especially around everyday, normal sounds. Like tinnitus, hyperacusis can be accompanied by anxiety disorders and major depression. As previously mentioned, phonophobia may be present as well. For these patients, antidepressants and anti anxiety medications as well as psychological counseling may be warranted.

Treatment of Diplacusis and Recruitment

Like hyperacusis, the treatment options for diplacusis and recruitment are limited. Fortunately, they rarely are in need of treatment, except in the case of the musician with MIHL in which the problem is interfering with his ability to perform. However, unlike in hyperacusis, the treatment of diplacusis employs the use of hearing protection devices. They can lower the overall sound level, bringing one down lower on the associated psychophysical tuning curve, so that the lowering of the perceived tone is minimized. Depending on the musical instrument, the appropriate device may alleviate the problem (Chasin, 1996). Occasional claims of success in the treatment of diplacusis and recruitment with TRT have been made, but these are very few in number. Interestingly, there is a report (Cherry & Brown, 1996) of one musician with intolerable diplacusis (and hyperacusis) in a deafened ear who was cured by surgical cochlear labyrinthectomy.

KEY POINT

Prevention of these disorders is of the utmost importance to insure the otologic health and the occupational longevity of a musician. The otolaryngologist must be able to recommend appropriate means of prevention, including high fidelity hearing protection devices, environmental modifications, and medical therapy when deemed necessary

SUMMARY

Like professional athletes, performing artists (especially musicians) develop medical maladies frequently associated with the risks of their profession. Physicians involved with performing arts medicine are quite familiar with the evaluation and treatment of the disorders of minor muscle groups that can befall on the musician. Just as important (but perhaps not as well recognized) are the multiple medical concerns for the health of the musician's otologic apparatus from chronic loud music exposure and how to properly address them. Disorders arising from NIOD exist among musicians and, if left unrecognized, can become a severe impairment. Therefore, it is essential that all otolaryngologists examining musicians are aware of its existence, be able to diagnose its presence, provide appropriate treatment and counseling, and educate as to means of prevention.

REFERENCES

Axelsson, A., & Lindgren, F. (1978). Hearing in pop musicians. *Acta Otolaryngologica*, *85*, 225-231.

Axelsson, A., & Lindgren, F. (1981). Hearing in classical musicians. *Acta Otolaryngologica* (Suppl. 377); 3-74.

Chasin, M. (1996). *Musicians and the prevention of hearing loss*. San Diego, CA: Singular.

Cherry, J. R., & Brown, M. J. (1996). Relief of severe hyperacusis and diplacusis in a deafened ear by cochlear labyrinthectomy. *Journal of Laryngology and Otology*, *110*(1), 57-58.

Chesky, K., & Henoch, M. A. (2000). Instrument-specific reports of hearing loss: Differences between classical and nonclassical musicians. *Medical Problems of Performing Artists*, *15*(1), 35-38.

Dey, F. L. (1970). Auditory fatigue and predicted permanent hearing defects from rock and roll music. *New England Journal of Medicine*, *282*(9), 467-470.

Fechter, L. D., Cheng, D., & Rao, D. (2002). Chemical asphyxiants and noise. *Noise Health*, *4*, 49-61.

Golz, A., Westerman, S. T., Westerman, L. M., Goldenberg, D., Netzer, A., Wiedmyer, T., et al. (2001). The effects of noise on the vestibular system. *American Journal of Otolaryngology*, *22*(3), 190-196.

Gunderson, E., Moline, J., Catalano, (1997). Risks of developing noise-induced hearing loss in employees of urban music clubs. *American Journal of Industrial Medicine*, *31*, 75-79.

Hall, J. W., & Bulla, W. A. (1999). Assessment of music-induced auditory dysfunction. *The Hearing Review*, *6*(2), 20-27.

Hart, C. W., Geltman, C. L., Schupbach, J., & Santucci, M. (1987). The musician and occupational sound hazards. *Medical Problems of Performing Artists*, *2*(3), 22-25.

Jastreboff, P. J., Gray, W. C., & Gold, S. L. (1996). Neurophysiological approach to tinnitus patients. *American Journal of Otolog*, *17*, 236-240.

Jastreboff, P. J. & Jastreboff, M. (2003). Tinnitus retraining therapy for patients with tinnitus and decreased sound tolerance. *The Otolaryngology Clinics of North America*, *36*(2), 321-336.

Kahari, K., Zachau, G., Eklof, M., Sandsjo, L., & Moller, C. (2003). Assessment of hearing and hearing disorders in rock/jazz musicians. *International Journal of Audiology*, *42*(5), 279-288.

Karlsson, K., Lundquist, P. G., & Olaussen, T. (1983). The hearing of symphony orchestra musicians. *Scandinavian Audiology*, *12*, 257-264.

Laitinen, H. (2005). Factors affecting the use of hearing protectors among classical music players. *Noise Health*, *7*(26), 21-29.

Lonsbury-Martin, B. L., & Martin, G. K. (2005). Noise-induced hearing loss. In C. W. Cummings (Ed.), *Cummings: Otolaryngology: head and neck surgery* (4th ed., pp. 1150-1163). Philadelphia: Mosby.

Lynch, E. D., & Kil, J. (2005). Compounds for the prevention and treatment of noise-induced hearing loss. *Drugs Discovery Today*, *10*(19), 1291-1298.

Morata, T. C., & Little, M. B. (2002). Suggested guidelines for studying the combined effects of occupational exposure to noise and chemicals on hearing. *Noise Health*, *4*, 73-87.

National Institutes of Health, Office of Medical Applications of Research. (1990). Consensus Conference on Noise and Hearing Loss. *Journal of the American Medical Association, 263*, 3185-3190.

Ostri, B. N., Eller, N., Dahlin, E., & Skylv, G. (1989). Hearing impairment in orchestral musicians. *Scandinavian Audiology, 18*(4), 243-249.

Sataloff, R. T. (1991). Hearing loss in musicians. *American Journal of Otology, 12*(2), 122-127.

Seidman, M. D., Jacobson, G. P. Update on tinnitus. (1996). *The Otolaryngologic Clinics of North America*. (pp. 455-465. Philadelphia: W.B. Saunders.

Shiley, S. G., Folmer, R. L., & McMenomey, S. O. (2005). Tinnitus and hyperacusis. In C. W. Cummings (Ed.), *Cummings: Otolaryngology: Head and neck surgery* (4th ed., pp. 1113-1126). Philadelphia: Mosby.

Shupak, A., Bar-El, E., Podoshin, L., Spitzer, O., Gordon, C. R., & Ben-David, J. (1994). Vestibular findings associated with chronic noise induced hearing impairment. *Acta Otolaryngologica 114*(6), 579-585.

Westmore, G. A., & Eversden, I. D. (1981). Noise-induced hearing loss and orchestral musicians. *Archives of Otolaryngology, 107*, 761-764.

Ylikoski, J., Juntunen, J., Matikainen, E., Ylikoski, M., & Ojala, M. (1988). Subclinical vestibular pathology in patients with noise-induced hearing loss from intense impulse noise. *Acta Otolaryngologica, 105*, 558-563.

4 Tinnitus, Hyperacusis, and Music

BY RICHARD S. TYLER, SON-A CHANG, PAN TAO,
STEPHANIE GOGEL, AND ANNE K. GEHRINGER

WHAT IS TINNITUS?

Tinnitus is the perception of sound in the absence of an external sound. It is commonly associated with noise induced hearing loss. There are two broad types of tinnitus. Middle-ear tinnitus is a result of abnormal blood vessels or muscle twitching in the middle ear cavity behind the eardrum. Sensorineural tinnitus involves the cochlea and/or auditory nervous system. Music induced tinnitus is one type of sensorineural tinnitus.

The most common descriptions of tinnitus include "ringing," "buzzing," "crickets," and "hissing" (Stouffer & Tyler, 1990). It can be constant or intermittent, can occur in one or both ears, and can vary its qualities from day to day. Tinnitus is a relatively common symptom in the general population. About 0.5% of the general population report tinnitus having a severe effect on their ability to lead a normal life (Coles, 1984). Its prevalence increases with age and with noise exposure. Tinnitus is now being seen more frequently in young people who are exposed to intense music for long periods of time.

People with tinnitus often report strong emotional reactions (including anxiety and depression). Tinnitus can also interfere with your hearing (including your perception of music). One of the more common complaints is getting to sleep at night, which can affect overall performance the next day. It is also associated with concentration difficulties, for example, when you are trying to learn a new musical tune or other complex task.

KEY POINT

About 0.5% of the general population report tinnitus having a severe effect on their ability to lead a normal life (Coles, 1984). It is a symptom and not a disease.

If a person listens to (or plays) intense music, tinnitus might be induced. Those exposed to modern and classical music are in danger of musically induced tinnitus. Data are accumulating to document the presence of music induced tinnitus (Bradley, Fortnum, & Coles, 1987;

Coelho, Sanchez, & Tyler, 2007a, b; Mercier, Luy, & Hohmann, 2003; Schmuziger, Patscheke, & Probst, 2006).

WHAT CAUSES TINNITUS?

Tinnitus is not a disease, but a symptom. It has several different causes and in many situations the precise cause is unknown. Generally speaking, the same factors that cause hearing loss can also cause tinnitus.

Noise Exposure

Noise induced hearing loss and noise induced tinnitus often go hand in hand. The most common situations causing noise induced tinnitus are working in noisy industries (like in manufacturing) or shooting guns. From our clinical experience, working in a noisy factory for only 2 or 3 years can cause tinnitus. Often, the tinnitus begins to appear only at the end of a shift and then later fades. Then, over months, it persists until it is a constant sound. Sometimes, tinnitus arises after a person has ended his or her exposure to noise, perhaps even months later. Gunshot induced tinnitus can sometimes occur after a single shot, but it is more common to develop after months or years of being exposed to gunfire.

Like hearing loss, there are primarily three factors that contribute to noise-induced tinnitus. The first factor is the noise level. The higher the noise level, the more likely a person will get tinnitus. Second is the duration of noise exposure. The longer the duration of the exposure, the more likely a person will get noise induced tinnitus. Having brief periods of rest (quiet periods) between episodes

of noise exposure will likely reduce the chance of noise induced tinnitus. Third is the presence of impulses (rapid bursts of high amplitude sound) (Axelsson & Prasher, 2000). The presence of impulses in a sound is known to make the sound more hazardous to your hearing.

> ### KEY POINT
>
> Three factors that contribute to noise induced tinnitus are noise level, duration of the noise, and the presence of impulses.

Guidelines for noise induced hearing loss can be applied to noise induced tinnitus. However, it should be remembered that these are only general guidelines, and there are critical individual differences. Some of us are more susceptible to noise induced hearing loss and tinnitus than others!

Music Exposure

Music can cause hearing loss and tinnitus just like noise. The same basic principles are involved. The higher the music levels and the longer the exposure, the greater the likelihood of music induced hearing loss and tinnitus. Music that includes impulsive sounds (such as those produced by cymbals or the rapid onset of horns) adds to the danger of music induced hearing loss and tinnitus.

Aging

All of us will eventually acquire a hearing loss as a result of aging (presbycusis). For some, this begins at 50 years of age, for others it might not start until age 70. Age-induced tinnitus likely follows a similar time course.

Other Causes

As we mentioned, most factors that cause hearing loss can cause tinnitus. However, tinnitus in some situations can be an important symptom of some other disease in its early stage. Because of this, if you develop tinnitus you should see an audiologist and an otologist. We review now a few other common causes.

Ménière's Disease

The typical symptoms of Ménière's disease include spells of dizziness, fluctuating hearing loss, and tinnitus. The treatments include medications, special diets, and sometimes surgery.

Acoustic Tumor

Although rare, it is important to determine if you have an acoustic neuroma (also known as vestibular schwannoma). Acoustic neuromas are nonmalignant tumors of the hearing nerve that are associated with an asymmetrical hearing loss, and patients often have unilateral tinnitus as the first symptom.

Medication

Tinnitus can also arise as a side effect of medication: there are over 300 prescription and nonprescription drugs that list tinnitus as a side effect. For example, aspirin, the "mycin" drugs, and quinine are associated with tinnitus. Stopping or altering the dose of some medications can reverse tinnitus. Check with your physician before making any changes to medications you may be taking (see Perry & Gantz, 2000).

KEY POINT

There are over 300 prescription and nonprescription drugs that list tinnitus as a side effect.

PREVENTING TINNITUS

Preventing music induced hearing loss is the best way to prevent music induced tinnitus. This includes reducing the level and duration of the music you listen to. You can lower the level of music by:

- Reducing the levels of music produced
- Putting distance between you and the music source
- Isolating yourself from the music (putting barriers between you and the music)
- Using hearing protection

Having periods of rest during long periods of music exposure will also reduce the likelihood of music induced tinnitus.

If you consider yourself at risk for music induced tinnitus, measure the noise levels, keep track of the duration of exposures, and determine whether you are exposed to impulsive noises. Noise levels you are exposed to can be measured with a sound level meter. The U.S. Department of Labor Occupational Safety and Health Administration suggests guidelines to reduce the likelihood of occupational noise induced hearing loss (OSHA,

1910.95). Continuous noise (similar to what would be present in many factories) that lasts 8 hours a day for 5 days a week at 80 to 85 dBA should be "safe" for most (but perhaps not all!). Furthermore, these guidelines do not consider impulsive noise or music.

Keep in mind these guidelines for preventing tinnitus are not based on musicians who might be exposed to high levels of music for shorter or longer periods of time. Tinnitus is a frequent complaint of classical music students who practice more than 20 hours per week (Hagberg, Thiringer, & Brandstrom, 2005).

Musicians can wear earplugs and earmuffs to decrease the sound levels. Typically, these are more effective at reducing the high frequency sounds than the low frequencies. One side effect of this is that the overall quality of the sound is altered, and this may be highly undesirable for musicians. Musicians' earplugs were designed to provide an equal amount of attenuation across the audible frequency range. This results in a more normal quality of sound, at the expense of being less effective at protection from noise and music. Noise cancellation headphones work extremely well when the external noise source is constant, such as with the noise from a continuous machine or an airplane engine. They are least effective for music, which is often changing in frequency and level.

Musicians can effectively use earmuff-headphone combination systems. A microphone (or direct electrical connection) transmits the signal (e.g., the music) to the headphones and a volume control allows the wearer to control the signal level. At the same time, the earmuffs reduce the external sound (perhaps the desired signal) plus some unwanted noise.

Laitinen (2005) reported that only 6% of musicians from five orchestras reported always using hearing protection. Perhaps as a result of this, 31% reported a hearing loss, and even more (37%) reported a temporary tinnitus. About 16% reported permanent tinnitus.

TREATING TINNITUS AND THE REACTIONS TO TINNITUS

There is no cure for tinnitus. Several studies of drugs and various devices might claim success. Based on controlled studies replicated by other investigators, there is no cure for tinnitus. If you are persuaded by a report claiming to be a cure, you should consult with your audiologist or otologist.

There are numerous approaches to help you cope or accept the influence of tinnitus. Medications are effective for depression, anxiety, and sleep. There are numerous treatments referred to as counseling and sound therapy (see Tyler, 2006, for a detailed overview of many of these). Our own approach uses Tinnitus Activities Therapy (Tyler et al., 2006), which includes collaborative counseling and partial masking. It emphasizes four areas, depending on individual needs. These include thoughts and emotions, hearing, sleep, and concentration.

For the thoughts and emotions section, listening to the patient is the first step. It is important to begin the counseling by learning from the patient what his or her major concerns are. Next, the patients are provided information about hearing, hearing loss, tinnitus, and attention. Both the clinician and the patient discuss ways to make tinnitus less important. After these steps, it is feasible to look for the ways to change the patient's lifestyle to manage her tinnitus better.

KEY POINT

Based on controlled studies replicated by other investigators, there is no cure for tinnitus. There are numerous approaches to help you cope or accept the influence of tinnitus.

For the hearing section, an effort is made to alleviate some of the communication difficulties associated with hearing loss and with tinnitus. This should additionally reduce stress associated with hearing difficulties and therefore indirectly help with managing tinnitus.

Sleep disturbances are very common in tinnitus patients (McKenna, 2000; Tyler & Baker, 1983). Some patients report difficulty falling asleep, waking during the night, early awakening, or being tired during the day. Information is provided to enhance the understanding of normal sleep patterns and to explore factors that can affect sleep such as stress, environmental noise, and room temperature. Activities and practice include arranging the bedroom to promote sleep, avoidance of alcohol, smoking, and eating before bedtime, using background sound to reduce the prominence of tinnitus, and learning relaxation exercises. Bedside relaxing music is one way to help promote sleep in patients with tinnitus.

Concentration is also an important area in our tinnitus therapy. Again, information is provided about factors that can distract or help one to concentrate. Activities include practice controlling and shifting attention in adverse circumstances. Decreasing the prominence of the tinnitus and increasing attention to the task are practiced.

Sound therapy involves using background sounds (including music) to reduce the prominence or loudness of tinnitus. Sometimes patients hear the background sound and tinnitus (partial masking) and sometimes the sound totally masks the tinnitus (total masking; e.g., Folmer, Martin, Shi, & Edlefsen, 2006). The sounds often used in sound therapy include broadband noise heard as "sssshhhh," soft and light background music such as classical baroque or simple piano music, and sound produced particularly for relaxation or distraction (such as waves lapping against the shore or raindrops falling on leaves).

There are devices available to facilitate sound therapy. Hearing aids can be helpful for individuals whose hearing loss is sufficient enough to affect their ability to communicate. Hearing aids can also help tinnitus because they can amplify background sound, which may provide partial masking. Tinnitus maskers or noise generators are also available. They produce a "sssshhhh" broadband noise, and the level of the noise can be adjusted by the individual. There are also combination units that include a hearing aid and a noise generator. Nonwearable sound generators that produce waterfall or rain sounds (or other sounds including music) are also available.

There are two self-help books for tinnitus that you might want to consider (Henry & Wilson, 2002; Tyler, 2008). You can also easily find useful information from our Web site (http://www.uihealth care.com/depts/med/otolaryngology/clinics/tinnitus/index.html).

TINNITUS AS AN EARLY WARNING FOR MUSIC INDUCED HEARING LOSS

If you are reading this chapter and have only recently been hearing tinnitus, even if it is only transient tinnitus, beware!

Although it is not always the case, tinnitus can sometimes be the first sign of the beginning of a noise or music induced hearing loss. And most commonly, tinnitus is a permanent symptom. If you hear tinnitus after listening to music, take this as a warning that you are damaging your ears. In some individuals, tinnitus typically does not begin until after several years of noise exposure. In other individuals, the tinnitus appears to begin after the noise exposure is over!

If you hear tinnitus after a concert (or any music experience), it is a warning sign to you that that particular music experience is likely damaging your hearing. Change your listening habits immediately!

TINNITUS, MUSIC, AND MUSICIANS

Music and tinnitus are related in several ways. We have already noted that music can cause tinnitus and briefly mentioned that it also can be used as a treatment tool. In this section, we note that some patients actually report a musiclike tinnitus and that some noteworthy musicians have tinnitus; we provide more details about music used to treat tinnitus and some songs that have been written about tinnitus.

KEY POINT

If you hear tinnitus after a concert (or any music experience), it is a warning sign to you that that particular music experience is likely damaging your hearing. Change your listening habits immediately.

Tinnitus Heard as Music

Although tinnitus is usually described as ringing, buzzing, or humming, it can also be heard as music! You should think of this in two very different ways. First, auditory hallucinations often accompany mental illness (e.g., Gordon, 1997). Sometimes the hallucinations are music or voices. Schakenraad, Teunisse, and Olde Rikkert (2006) described the content of musical hallucinations. They listed children's songs, piano music, and other classical music as the most common content of musical hallucinations. Second, there are people who hear a musical tinnitus but do not have any mental illness. They report their tinnitus as sounding like parts of songs: sometimes instruments, sometimes singing. This is reasonable as it has been known for many years that electrical stimulation of the auditory area in the brain can result in hearing music (or voices). These people likely have a tinnitus that originates in the brain.

Musicians with Tinnitus

Depending on the definition, the prevalence of tinnitus in the normal population varies from about 1 to 15%. In musicians, however, one study reported that as many as 37% of musicians have had temporary tinnitus (Laitinen, 2005).

There are many well-known musicians and musical artists who have tinnitus. Barbra Streisand, Pete Townshend of The Who, and Liberty DeVitto, long-time drummer for Billy Joel, have all publicly acknowledged having tinnitus. An Internet search for "tinnitus and musicians" produces a long list of singers and performers who have tinnitus.

Not only modern loud rock music but also classical music can lead to tinnitus. Ludwig van Beethoven and Bedrich Smetana were musicians in the 1700s to 1800s that also reportedly had tinnitus and hearing loss (Morgenstern, 2005). However, the hazards of intense and continuous exposure to musical sounds may also threaten today's classical musicians as well. Rosanowski and Eysholdt (1996) reported on a musician who complained that one (but not the other) of his violins exacerbated his tinnitus.

Music Used to Treat Tinnitus

It may seem ironic that some music can relieve the symptoms of tinnitus when loud music also can cause it; however, music has been successfully applied in several therapeutic applications (Davis & Thaut, 1989; Standley, 1995). Music can be used to facilitate systematic desensitization to tinnitus by employing the dynamic nature of the music to intermittently mask the perception of tinnitus as well as to facilitate relaxation. If the brain is exposed to nonsignificant, low level music, it can habituate to it and it may interfere with the detection of the tinnitus signal by the brain. Many tinnitus sufferers have reported that they prefer to listen to music to partially mask their tinnitus (Davis, Wilde, & Steed, 2002a, 2002b; Kitahara, 1988; Seidel, 1991; Vernon & Schleuning, 1978). Al-Jassim (1988) asked 41 patients to rate 5-minute recordings of music, relaxation exercises, pure tone, or band noise. Of that sample, 88% ranked music as the most preferable sound.

Many tinnitus sufferers have reported that they prefer to listen to music to partially mask their tinnitus. Davis (2006) has developed a strategy whereby individually modified music and noise are combined to desensitize patients to their tinnitus. Tyler (Shafer, 2004) has suggested that clinicians need to be wary when using music therapy with experienced musicians. They are likely to analyze the music with a critical ear, and this can prevent them from relaxing enough to use the music as a therapy tool. However, music has potential advantages over noise and can be more easily put in the background for many.

Songs about Tinnitus

The dramatic impact that tinnitus can have is perhaps illustrated nowhere better than in the lyrics of songs written about tinnitus. In fact, some bands and musical titles either name or imply tinnitus.

This is illustrated in the work of Bedrich Smetana, a Czech composer, dating back to 1876 (Morgenstern, 2005). In his quartet, "Aus Meinem Leben" ("From My Life"), Smetana devoted a harmonic with a sustained chord into one of the movements of his piece. This appears to be a representation of his version of what he heard with his own tinnitus.

Many different musicians have even incorporated lyrics into some of their pieces describing their tinnitus. For example, U2's single "Staring at the Sun" (Bono and The Edge, 2000, track 6) contains lyrics leading one to believe that at least one member of the band suffers from tinnitus. The lyrics include:

"There's an insect in your ear

if you scratch it won't disappear"
(Bono and The Edge, 2000, track 6).

In addition to those listed here, there are many other musical lyrics as well as other creations, including poetry and written works, which appear to be inspired by the author or another individual dealing with tinnitus. A group of tinnitus sufferers from Brazil have written a play, with music and lyrics, about all the trials they have experienced because of their tinnitus (Figure 4–1).

HYPERACUSIS

Tinnitus and hearing loss can be accompanied by strong reactions to intense sounds, which is called hyperacusis. The terminology used for hyperacusis is not standardized, but we distinguish three forms (Table 4–1). If you perceive sounds as very loud that others would perceive as only moderately loud, you have loudness hyperacusis. If you are annoyed by sounds that are only moderately intense, you have annoyance hyperacusis. If you develop a fear of sounds, perhaps because

you believe they will be very loud or very annoying, you have fear hyperacusis (sometimes called phonophobia).

The same things we have said about the causes of tinnitus, preventing tinnitus, and treating tinnitus can also be said about hyperacusis.

Some people with hyperacusis use earplugs to reduce the level of even moderately intense sounds in everyday situations, but this is not recommended. Of course, we should all protect our hearing from intense sounds, but this use of earplugs in everyday situations does not relieve the hyperacusis when the earplugs are removed. In fact, wearing earplugs too frequently in everyday situations might even result in the auditory system becoming even more reactive to intense sounds or hyperacusic.

There are no cures for hyperacusis. It is sometimes treated with continuous low level noise, increasing dosages of noise during specified listening periods,

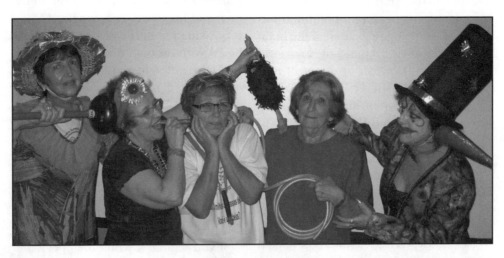

Figure 4–1. A tinnitus sufferer (*center*) looks forlorn as she is surrounded by "treatments," which include a plunger, a cigar, a black chicken, a water hose, and the sound devil (Brazilian group Dádiva in Rio, December 2007). (Photograph by Rich Tyler). Used with permission.

Table 4–1. The Forms of Hyperacusis	
Form of Hyperacusis	*Description*
Loudness hyperacusis	Sounds that are not loud for others are very loud for you.
Annoyance hyperacusis	You are annoyed by moderately intense sounds.
Fear hyperacusis	You become afraid of some sounds, perhaps even avoiding some situations.

and controlled listening to recorded sounds that evoke hyperacusis (see a review by Tyler, Oleson, Noble, Coelho, & Ji, 2007).

KEY POINT

Some people with hyperacusis use earplugs to reduce the level of even moderately intense sounds in everyday situations, but this is not recommended.

SUMMARY

Tinnitus is real; it is not a phantom sound. There is spontaneous neural activity in your hearing system that corresponds to the tinnitus you hear. Noise exposure, including music, is one of the most common causes. Keep in mind that tinnitus is a symptom; it has many causes and probably many mechanisms and will likely require many treatments. Tinnitus can be an early warning sign for noise induced hearing loss. Reducing noise exposure will help prevent noise induced tinnitus. Currently, there is no cure for tinnitus. However, counseling and sound therapies can be very helpful in managing tinnitus.

Acknowledgments. We wish to acknowledge grant support provided by the National Institutes of Health (NIH Grant 5R01DC005972-02). Richard Tyler is a consultant for Neuromonics Inc.

REFERENCES

Al-Jassim, A. (1988). The use of Walkman Mini-stereo system as a tinnitus masker. *Journal of Laryngology and Otology*, *102(1)*, 27–28.

Axelsson, A., & Prasher, D. (2000). Tinnitus induced by occupational and leisure noise. *Noise Health*, *8*, 47–54.

Bradley, R., Fortnum, H., & Coles, R. (1987). Patterns of exposure of school children to amplified music. *British Journal of Audiology*, *21(2)*, 119–125.

Coelho, C., Sanchez, T., & Tyler, R. (2007). Hyperacusis, sound annoyance, and loudness hypersensitivity in children. *Progress in Brain Research*, *166*, 169–178.

Coelho, C., Sanchez, T. G., & Tyler, R. S. (2007). Tinnitus in children and associated risk factors. *Progress in Brain Research*, *166*, 179–194.

Coles, R. (1984). Epidemiology of tinnitus: 1. Prevalence. *Journal of Laryngology and Otology*, (Suppl. 9), 7–15.

Davis, P. B. (2006). Music and the acoustic desensitization protocol for tinnitus. In

R. S. Tyler (Ed.), *Tinnitus treatment: Clinical protocols* (pp. 146–160). New York: Thieme Medical.

Davis, P. B., & Thaut, M. H. (1989). The influence of preferred relaxing music on measures of state anxiety, relaxation, and physiological responses. *Music Therapy, 26*(4), 168–187.

Davis, P. B., Wilde, R. A., & Steed, L. G. (2002a). A habituation-based rehabilitation technique using the Acoustic Desensitisation Protocol. *Seventh International Tinnitus Seminar*, 188–191.

Davis, P. B., Wilde, R. A., & Steed, L. G. (2002a). Clinical trial findings of the Acoustic Desensitisation Protocol: A habituation-based rehabilitation technique. *Seventh International Tinnitus Seminar*, 74–77.

Folmer, R., Martin, W., Shi, Y., & Edlefsen, L. (2006). Tinnitus sound therapies. In R. S. Tyler (Ed.), *Tinnitus treatment: Clinical protocols* (pp. 176–186). New York: Thieme.

Gordon, A. (1997). Do musical hallucinations always arise from the inner ear? *Medical Hypotheses, 49*, 111–122.

Hagberg, M., Thiringer, G., & Brandstrom, L. (2005). Incidence of tinnitus, impaired hearing and musculoskeletal disorders among students enrolled in academic music education—A retrospective cohort study. *International Archives of Occupational and Environmental Health, 78*, 575–583.

Henry, J., & Wilson, P. (2002). *Tinnitus: A self-management guide for the ringing in your ears*. Boston: Allyn and Bacon.

Kitahara, M. (1988). Tinnitus: *Pathophysiology and management*. Tokyo: Igaku-Shoin Medical.

Laitinen, H. (2005). Factors affecting the use of hearing protectors among classical music players. *Noise Health, 7*(26), 21–29.

McKenna, L. (2000). Tinnitus and insomnia. In R. S. Tyler (Ed.), *Tinnitus handbook* (pp. 59–84). San Diego, CA: Singular.

Mercier, V., Luy, D., & Hohmann, B. (2003). The sound exposure of the audience at a music festival. *Noise Health, 5*(19), 51–58.

Morgenstern, L. (2005). The bells are ringing. *Perspectives in Biology and Medicine, 48*, 396–407.

Perry, B. P., & Gantz, B. J. (2000). Medical and surgical evaluation and management of tinnitus. In R. S. Tyler (Ed.), *Tinnitus handbook* (pp. 221–241). San Diego, CA: Singular.

Rosanowski, F., & Eysholdt, U. (1996). In situ sound pressure measurement in a professional violinist with bilateral tinnitus. *Laryngorhinootologie, 75*(9), 514–516.

Schakenraad, S., Teunisse, R., & Olde Rikkert, M. (2006). Musical hallucinations in psychiatric patients. *International Journal of Geriatric Psychiatry 21*, 394–397.

Schmuziger, N., Patscheke, J., & Probst, R. (2006). Hearing in nonprofessional pop/rock musicians. *Ear and Hearing, 27*(4), 321–330.

Seidel, S. J. (1991). A hierarchy for tinnitus patient management. In J.-M. Aran & R. Dauman (Eds.), *Proceedings of the Fourth International Tinnitus Seminar* (pp. 497–499). Amsterdam/New York: Kugler.

Shafer, D. (2004, November 2). Music studied as tinnitus relief. *AHSA Leader*, pp. 1, 14.

Standley, J. (1995). Music as a therapeutic intervention in medical/dental treatment: Research and clinical applications. In T. Wigram, B. Saperston, & R. West (Eds.), *The art and science of music therapy: A handbook* (pp. 3–22). Chur, Switzerland: Harwood Academic.

Stouffer, J. L., & Tyler, R. S. (1990). Characterization of tinnitus by tinnitus patients. *Journal of Speech and Hearing Disorders, 55*, 439.

Tyler, R. (2006). Neurophysiological models, psychological models, and treatments for tinnitus. In R. S. Tyler (Ed.), *Tinnitus treatment: Clinical protocols* (pp. 1–22). New York: Thieme.

Tyler, R. S. (Ed.). (2008). *The consumer handbook on tinnitus*. Sedona, AZ: Auricle.

Tyler, R., & Baker, L. (1983). Difficulties experienced by tinnitus sufferers. *Journal of Speech and Hearing Disorders, 48*, 150–154.

Tyler, R. S., Gehringer, A. K., Noble, W., Dunn, C. C., Witt, S. A., & Bardia, A. (2006). Tinnitus activities treatment. In R. S. Tyler (Ed.), *Tinnitus treatment: Clinical protocols* (pp. 116-131). New York: Thieme.

Tyler, R. S., Noble, W., Coelho, C., Haskell, G., & Bardia, A. (in press). Tinnitus and hyperacusis. In J. Katz, R. Burkard, L. Medwetsky, & L. Hood (Eds.), *Handbook of clinical audiology* (6th ed.). Baltimore: Lippincott Williams & Wilkins.

Tyler, R. S., Oleson, J., Noble, W., Coelho, C., & Ji, H. (2007). Clinical trials for tinnitus: Study populations, designs, measurement variables, and data analysis. *Progress in Brain Research, 166,* 499-509.

U.S. Department of Labor Occupational Safety and Health Administration. (n.d.). *Regulations (standards-29 CFR) occupational noise exposure. 1910.95.* Retrieved November 30, 2007, from http://www.osha.gov/pls/oshaweb/owadisp.show_document?p_table=STANDARDS&p_id=9735

Bono and The Edge. (2000). Staring at the sun [Recorded by U2]. On *Hasta la vista baby* [CD]. Mexico City: Polygram International Publishing BV. (December 3, 1997)

Vernon, J., & Schleuning, A. (1978). Tinnitus: A new management. *Laryngoscope, 88*(3), 413-419.

5 Do Headphones Cause Hearing Loss?

Risk of Music Induced Hearing Loss for the Music Consumer

BY BRIAN J. FLIGOR

NATURE OF THE PROBLEM

Increasing population densities and human encroachment in previously uninhabited areas have served to continually increase sound levels in society. Noise is now virtually everywhere. According to Berger (2003), 40% of the European community is continuously exposed to transportation noise of 55 dBA (similar to a normal voice in the background) and 20% are exposed to greater than 65 dBA (similar to a voice at a conversational distance). This level of 65 dBA is considered by the World Health Organization to be intrusive or annoying (World Health Organization [WHO], 1995). Of the 20 locations in Washington State that nature recordist, Gordon Hempton, reported to be "noise-free" in 1984, only three locations remained noise-free in 1989 (Grossmann, 1995). In the United States workforce, an estimated 30 million people are regularly exposed to sound levels in excess of 85 dBA, which is considered the thresh-old for a hazardous sound exposure (National Institute for Occupational Safety and Health [NIOSH], 1998). Of the 31 million Americans with hearing loss, it is estimated that 10 million of these are at least in part a result of noise (National Institutes of Health [NIH], 1990).

With the ever-increasing din of society intruding on a person's peaceful space (and healthy hearing), people have fought back by controlling their own soundscapes. If they cannot control the unwanted environmental noise, they can mask it by presenting to their ears a desired sound at a level sufficient to perceptually mask the unwanted noise. Car stereos, home theaters, books on tape, podcasts, and portable music content presented via earphones are extraordinarily popular. The ubiquitous Apple iPod and other portable digital music players clearly met a need for people to build their own soundscapes wherever they go. Unfortunately, while the brain may make the distinction between wanted and unwanted sound, the ear does not, and without ever giving the ear time to rest and recover from excessive sound levels, the sensory cells in the inner ear eventually are exhausted and die. Consequently, ears age prematurely and we lose our gift of exquisitely fine hearing at a younger age.

Music "Consumption"

Although a focus of this book is to consider music as a form of occupational noise exposure in the performing musician, the musician's sound exposure is certainly not limited to practice or performance. Musicians may be the most adamant consumers of others' musical performance (live or recorded), so off-the-job exposures ought to be factored into the overall consideration of risk for noise induced hearing loss. Within the general population are those who, although not musicians themselves, truly *consume* music. Most published studies of duration of headphone use report average weekly use of only a few hours in cassette players and compact disc (CD) players (Felchlin, Hohmann, & Matefi, 1998; Meyer-Bisch, 1996), and possibly longer average weekly use with digital music players (Zogby, 2006). However, in each study, there are outliers who use headphones for much greater periods of time. Felchlin et al, 1998, reported 10% of headphone users in their study listened longer than 10 hours per week, and Ahmed et al. (2007) reported 5% of their subjects used portable digital music players for 4 to 8 hours per session and as often as 7 days per week.

Music has even been conceptualized as having commonalities with acknowledged addictive substances such as alcohol and nicotine. Florentine, Hunter, Robinson, Ballou, and Buus (1998) devel-

oped a 32-item screening instrument, adapted to apply to music listening from the Michigan Alcoholism Screening Test (a well-known, sensitive questionnaire used to screen for alcoholism), to screen for maladaptive music listening behavior. Although the impact of music addiction may be less problematic than alcohol or drug addiction, the Florentine et al. (1998) study did identify individuals who exhibited addiction-like behavior, such as withdrawal when deprived of loud music and a need to continue listening to loud music despite knowing that they had a music induced hearing loss.

CAN USING HEADPHONES TO LISTEN TO MUSIC REALLY CAUSE A MUSIC INDUCED HEARING LOSS?

Older Technology: Cassette Tape Players and CD Players

Whether or not hearing loss from using headphones should be a public health concern continues to be a matter of debate. Some authors have suggested that 5 to 10% of headphone users are at risk for noise induced hearing loss (Clark, 1991), whereas others suggest a much smaller number are truly at risk (Rice, Rossi, & Olina, 1987; Turunen-Rise, Flottorp, & Tvete, 1991). However, it is not in doubt that each generation of portable music player (cassette player, CD player, and hard disk/flash memory music player) produces levels of 100 decibels or higher. Early studies investigating hearing loss risk from cassette players reported maximum output levels of 124 dBA (Wood & Lipscomb, 1972) and 110 to 128 dBA (Katz, Gertsman, Sanderson,

& Buchanan, 1982). The reported output of the cassette players in the Katz et al. (1982) study exceeded 85 dBA at 30% of the volume control. There are concerns the methodology employed in these two early studies does not allow for direct comparison to established damage risk criteria because they did not report free-field or diffuse-field equivalent sound pressure levels (International Organisation for Standardisation [ISO] 11904-2, 2004); nonetheless, the reported levels raised considerable concern. Turunen-Rise et al. (1991) reported free-field equivalent sound levels from cassette players of 98 to 108 dBA and from CD players of 98 to 110 dBA at the highest volume control settings. In this study, six subjects exhibited a temporary threshold shift (TTS) after listening to music at 80% of the maximum volume setting on cassette player for 1 hour. Although one might consider these results to suggest using headphones poses a risk to the user's hearing, Turunen-Rise et al. (1991) interpreted their findings conservatively; they concluded there was little risk for permanent hearing loss as the median TTS was 12 dB (not considered a large shift), and the six subjects (seated in a quiet laboratory) reported 80% volume control setting was higher than they would have preferred.

KEY POINT

Headphones can be used at levels and for durations that pose a risk for permanent hearing loss. Although the majority of headphone users are not at risk for significant noise induced hearing loss, a small but significant percent of users may develop noise induced hearing loss, given listening levels and durations.

Fligor and Cox (2004) reported the output levels from commercially available CD players and after-market accessory headphones. Figure 5-1 (from Fligor & Cox, 2004) shows the free-field equivalent output levels as a function of volume control (each number of the abscissa corresponds to the decade percent of volume control; for example, "5" equals 50% of the maximum volume control). A few headphone-CD player combinations achieved sound levels exceeding 120 dBA free-field equivalent, and peak sound pressure levels above 130 dB SPL, depending on music genre. Using a conservative damage risk criterion (NIOSH, 1998), the authors suggested limiting listening level to 60% of the maximum volume control if listening for 1 hour or less per day, and using headphones that were purchased with the CD player, to reduce risk for music induced hearing loss.

Newer Technology: Portable Digital Music Players

Williams (2005) investigated chosen listening levels in passers-by on a busy city street in urban Australia. Although the focus of that study was not to determine sound levels from portable digital music players, it can be surmised from the results that levels from portable digital music players exceeded 100 dBA free-field equivalent. Ahmed et al. (2007) reported levels from the Apple iPod earbud earphones depended on the music genre and graphic equalizer setting, but at maximum volume control, free-field equivalent sound levels approached 100 dBA. French law mandates a maximum level of 100 dB from personal stereo systems with headphones and specifies a maximum

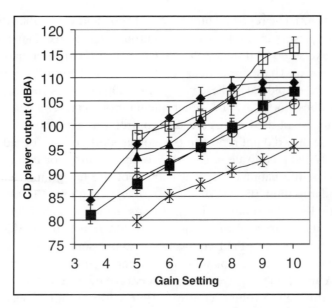

Figure 5–1. Average free-field equivalent output level for six commercially available CD players, across headphones used in the study. Recordings were made at gain (volume control) settings 5–10, including Automatic Volume Limiting System (AVLS) on the Sony systems (corresponding to level 3.5). Error bars represent the standard deviation across the different headphones. *Note.* From "Output Levels of Commercially Available Portable Compact Disk Players and the Potential Risk to Hearing," by B. J. Fligor & L. C. Cox, 2004, *Ear and Hearing, 25*, pp. 513-527. Used with permission.

output voltage to headphones not exceed 150 millivolts (Legifrance, 2005).

Preliminary findings from ongoing studies of output levels from portable digital music players have been presented by this author at national meetings (Portnuff & Fligor, 2006). To date, our findings are in good agreement with those of Williams (2005) and Ahmed et al. (2007). Further, similar to Fligor and Cox (2004), a rough "acoustic speed limit" for using headphones in a manner that reduces risk for music induced hearing loss, volume control should be limited to 80% of maximum if listening duration is 90 min-

utes or less per day, using earphones that are purchased with the portable digital music player.

It should be noted that simply because headphones can be driven to levels that pose a risk to hearing, that does not mean people actually use headphones in a manner that poses a hazard. Fligor and Cox (2004) observed and Portnuff and Fligor (2006) have reported that headphones positioned in the ear canal or directly over the ear canal have the capacity to achieve higher sound levels than headphones that sit on top of the pinna (supra-aural) or surround the pinna (circumaural). Neither report investigated listening behavior, nor does evidence exist to date suggesting that listening behavior is affected by maximum output levels available. Listening behavior and headphone type will be considered in detail later in this chapter.

KEY POINT

The type of headphone influences the range of sound level (from softest to loudest), but there is no evidence that this dynamic range influences a person's chosen listening level.

THE INFLUENCE OF LISTENING ENVIRONMENT ON CHOSEN LISTENING LEVEL

Common sense dictates that if a desired signal is masked by an undesired signal, the desired signal's intensity can either be increased, or the undesired signal's intensity decreased. Many people have experienced surprise at the level of their car stereo when they reduce speed as they exit a highway, not realizing how high they had turned their music to overcome road noise. As noted in this chapter's introduction, the world is a noisy place. Often, ambient environmental noise cannot be easily controlled by the individual; if the individual is listening to music via headphones, high level ambient noise should induce the headphone user to increase the volume control.

Airo et al. (1996) reported chosen listening levels to headphones in quiet and in noisy environments. Mean free-field equivalent chosen listening level in quiet was 69 dBA, with 15% choosing levels in excess of 85 dBA. The mean chosen listening level was raised to 85 dBA when the background noise reached 72 dBA. In quiet environments, the majority (but not all) chose to listen at levels well below 85 dBA. When the noise level in the ambient environment began to interfere with music listening, subjects increased the volume, seeking on average a signal-to-noise ratio of +13 dB.

Williams (2005) surveyed the listening levels of 55 passers-by in Melbourne and Sydney, Australia, outside of busy public transportation hubs. The average ambient noise level was 73.2 dBA, and the average listening level was 86.1 dBA. Thus, as with the Airo et al. (1996) study, an average chosen signal-to-noise ratio of +13 dB was observed. A wide range was seen in their group, with chosen levels from 73.7 dBA to 110.2 dBA. Self-reported listening duration (in a given listening session as well as weekly listening habits) was also obtained, so that estimates of damage risk could be made. Available estimates of damage risk from using headphones will be discussed later in this chapter.

Preliminary findings from a manuscript currently in preparation have been presented describing the effect of ambient background noise as well as the influence of headphone type on chosen listening level (Fligor & Ives, 2006). In our study, subjects listened to music in various levels of background noise using earphones that provided varying amounts of passive sound isolation. Average chosen listening level in quiet was roughly 61 dBA across all headphones. As background noise increased, chosen listening level increased in a predictable fashion in those subjects who chose moderate levels in quiet. The majority of subjects chose levels 85 dBA or greater when listening in a simulated airplane cabin (80 dBA background noise) when using earphones that provided no sound isolation (an earbud and a supra-aural headphone). Using an earphone that provided considerable passive sound isolation, an ER-6i in-the-canal earphone, the number of subjects who chose a listening level of 85 dBA or greater decreased dramatically.

KEY POINT

In quiet, the type of headphone has little bearing on chosen listening level. As the level of noise in the listening environment increases, people turn their music louder. The amount they increase the volume depends on the amount of acoustic isolation provided by the earphone. The more sound isolation, the less ambient noise affects chosen listening level.

AVAILABLE EVIDENCE THAT LISTENING TO MUSIC VIA HEADPHONES POSES A HAZARD

Evidence that listening to music via headphones poses a risk to hearing is sparse. As it is, risk is a relative term, with maximum permissible exposure levels varying depending on the purpose of the damage risk application. For instance, the Occupational Safety and Health Administration (OSHA) (1983) promulgates regulations governing noise exposure in occupational sectors that allow a maximum permissible exposure level of 90 dBA for an 8-hour time weighted average (TWA), using a 5 dB time-intensity trading ratio (exchange rate). Following this maximum permissible exposure level of 90 dBA TWA, 22% of exposed persons would still sustain a significant noise induced hearing loss after a 40-year working lifetime (Prince, Stayner, Smith, & Gilbert, 1997).

REPORTED HEARING DAMAGE FROM HEADPHONE USE

Actual cases of confirmed noise induced hearing loss from headphone listening are few. Meyer-Bisch (1996) conducted high resolution pure-tone audiometry on a huge study population and stratified subjects into those who used personal cassette players (PCPs) longer than 7 hours per week and those who used PCPs 2 to 7 hours per week. No attempt was made to assess chosen listening levels. A very small, but statistically significant, elevation of pure-tone thresholds was seen in the PCP users who listened for at least 7 hours weekly, compared to those who used a PCP for shorter durations.

LePage and Murray (1998) conducted transient evoked otoacoustic emissions (TEOAEs) measures on 1724 patients, and stratified subjects into four categories: non-noise exposed, exposed to industrial noise only, personal stereo system users with no industrial noise exposure, and personal stereo system users who were also exposed to industrial noise. Relative to the control group (non-noise exposed), TEOAE response was, on average, reduced in both personal stereo system users and in those exposed to industrial noise only, and an additive effect on TEOAE reduction was observed in those exposed to both industrial noise and personal stereo systems. Multiple linear regression modeling showed that "heavy" personal stereo system use had a greater effect on reduction of TEOAE response than did industrial noise exposure.

Time-Weighted Average Estimates

Despite the uncertainty that damage risk criteria should apply to music exposures in a manner equivalent to industrial noise exposures, a few studies have estimated time-weighted averages based on measured chosen listening levels and reported listening duration and frequency of use. Felchlin et al. (1998) reported a mean listening duration of 4 hours per week (range 1 to 21 hours) in 350 users of personal cassette players. Average listening level was 83 dBA and two fifths chose levels greater than 85 dBA. There was no correlation between cumulative listening duration and chosen listening level. The average estimated noise exposure was 72 dBA TWA, with 10% estimated to exceed 85 dBA TWA, and 5% exceeding 87 dBA TWA.

Rice et al. (1987) surveyed headphone listening time in 500 school children (average age 15.7 years) and conducted listening level measurements in a subset of subjects. They estimated that 5% of subjects in their study would meet or exceed a TWA of 90 dBA. To consider whether or not such exposure might result in a *hearing disability* Rice et al. (1987) compared their estimates of noise exposure to models predicting noise induced permanent threshold shift. Defining hearing disability as equal to or greater

than 30 dB HL averaged across 1000, 2000, and 3000 Hz, only 0.065% would have a hearing disability (one in 1538 headphone users). This estimate of a very small percentage of population risk could be misleading. Their definition of hearing disability is very liberal; a *material hearing impairment* (which OSHA, 1983, seeks to limit to not more than 22% of the exposed population) is a weighted average across 1000, 2000, 3000, and 4000 Hz of 25 dB HL. If Rice et al. (1987) had used the OSHA material hearing impairment definition for hearing disability, a much higher percentage would have been found to be at risk.

The subjects in Williams (2005) were users of portable digital music players, which might suggest that longer listening time would be seen (and correspondingly higher TWA), compared to studies of cassette player use. Williams (2005) conducted his study in what was considered a "worse-case scenario" where listening levels were obtained after a person had set the chosen level in fairly high background noise (ambient noise was an average 73.2 dBA). If measured chosen listening levels were typical, then based on self-reported listening duration and frequency, Williams (2005) estimated an average 79.8 dBA TWA in headphone users. Considering that this exposure is below the maximum permissible occupational exposure level of 85 dBA TWA in Australia, Williams (2005) reported that the average headphone user is not at risk for a music induced hearing loss. He noted, however, that his TWA estimate was above 75 dBA TWA (considered the maximum level for negligible noise induced hearing loss risk); 24% of his subjects had an estimated 85 dBA TWA or greater, and 3% had 100 dBA TWA or greater.

KEY POINT

Being able to hear users' music from their headphones does not mean they are at risk for music induced hearing loss. *Not* being able to hear a user's music does not mean he is listening at "safe" levels.

KEY POINT

Directed education and reasonable technological interventions would be useful for reducing the risk for music induced hearing loss in consumers.

SUMMARY

Data are available confirming all generations of portable music players produce levels that can cause music induced hearing loss, should the user choose to listen at high volume control settings for sufficient durations. It is necessary that headphones achieve at least moderately high sound levels when necessary. Discussing the issue with Dr. Mead Killion of Etymotic Research, Inc., Elk Grove Village, IL, he said "You wouldn't want a car with a speed limit governor set at 55 miles per hour!" (M. Killion, personal communication, April 21, 2004).

Studies assessing listening behavior indicate that a small but significant percent of people chose listening levels that put them at risk for permanent hearing loss. Hearing loss from high level music exposure is subtle, starting in high frequencies before affecting lower frequencies, making the hearing loss obvious.

Hearing loss from all high level sound is cumulative over one's lifetime, so the amount of hearing loss contribution from a single source (like headphone use) would be exceedingly difficult to pinpoint. Consequently, *proof* that headphones cause hearing loss in a large percentage of the population will not be forthcoming, so it is incumbent upon the hearing health professional and the consumer to arm themselves with knowledge, and in some cases, reasonable technological interventions to assist in minimizing the potential risk for music induced hearing loss.

REFERENCES

Ahmed, S., Fallah, S., Garrido, B., King, M., Morrish, T., Pereira, D., et al. (2007). Use of portable audio devices by university students. *Canadian Acoustics, 35*(1), 35-52.

Airo, E., Pekkarinen, J., & Olkinuora, P. (1996). Listening to music with headphones: An assessment of noise exposure. *Acustica, 82*, 885-894.

Berger, E. H. (2003). Noise control and hearing conservation: Why do it? In E. H. Berger, L. H. Royster, J. D. Royster, D. P. Driscoll, & M. Layne (Eds.), *The noise manual* (5th ed., pp. 2-17). Fairfax, VA: American Industrial Hygiene Association.

Clark, W. W. (1991). Noise exposure from leisure activities: A review. *Journal of the Acoustical Society of America, 90*(1), 175-181.

Felchlin, I., Hohmann, B. W., & Matefi, L. (1998). Personal cassette players: A hazard to hearing? In D. Prasher, L. Luxon, & I. Pyykko (Eds.), *Advances in noise research: Vol. 2. Protection against noise* (pp. 95-100). London: Whurr.

Fligor, B. J., & Cox, L. C. (2004). Output levels of commercially available portable compact disk players and the potential risk to hearing. *Ear and Hearing, 25*, 513-527.

Fligor, B. J., & Ives, T. E. (2006, October). *Does headphone type affect risk for recreational noise-induced hearing loss?* Paper presented at the NIHL in Children Meeting, Cincinnati, OH. Lay-paper retrieved December 31, 2007, from http://www.hearingconservation.org/docs/virtual PressRoom/FligorIves.pdf

Florentine, M., Hunter, W., Robinson, M., Ballou, M., & Buus, S. (1998). On the behavioral characteristics of loud-music listening. *Ear & Hearing, 19*(6), 420-428.

Grossmann, J. (1995, April). The sound of silence. *American Way,* 75-78, 114-116.

Katz, A. E., Gertsman, H. L., Sanderson, R. G., & Buchanan, R. (1982). Stereo earphones and hearing loss. *New England Journal of Medicine, 307,* 1460-1461.

International Organisation for Standardisation (ISO) 11904-2. (2004). *Acoustics: Determination of sound emission from sound sources placed close to the ear: Part 2. Technique using a manikin.* Geneva, Switzerland: ISO.

Legifrance. (2005). Arréte du 8 novembre 2005 portant application de l'article L. 5232-1 du code de la santé publique relatif aux baladeurs musicaux. *Journal Officiel de la République Française 301*(117), 20115.

LePage, E. L., & Murray, N. M. (1998). Latent cochlear damage in personal stereo users: A study based on click-evoked otoacoustic emissions. *Medical Journal of Australia. 169*(11-12), 588-592.

Meyer-Bisch, C. (1996). Epidemiological evaluation of hearing damage related to strongly amplified music (personal cassette players, discotheques, rock concerts): high-definition audiometric survey on 1364 subjects. *Audiology, 35,* 121-142.

National Institute for Occupational Safety and Health. (1998). *Criteria for a recommended standard: Occupational noise exposure, revised criteria.* Pub. No. 98-126. Cincinnati, OH: Author.

National Institutes of Health (NIH) Consensus Statement Noise and Hearing Loss. (1990).

Journal of the American Medical Association, 263, 3185-3190.

Occupational Safety and Health Administration. (1983). Occupational noise exposure: Hearing conservation amendment; Final rule. *Federal Register, 48,* 9738-9785.

Portnuff, C. D. F., & Fligor, B. J. (2006, October). *Sound output levels of the iPod and other MP3 players: Is there potential risk to hearing?* Paper presented at the NIHL in Children Meeting, Cincinnati, OH. Lay-paper retrieved December 31, 2007, from http://www.hearingconservation.org/docs/virtualPressRoom/portnuff.htm

Prince, M. M., Stayner, L. T., Smith, R. J., & Gilbert, S. J. (1997). A re-examination of risk estimates from the NIOSH Occupational Noise and Hearing Survey (ONHS). *Journal of the Acoustical Society of America, 101*(2), 950-963.

Rice, C. G., Rossi, G., & Olina, M. (1987). Damage risk from personal cassette players. *British Journal of Audiology, 21,* 279-288.

Turunen-Rise, I., Flottorp, G., & Tvete, O. (1991). Personal cassette players ('Walkman'). Do they cause noise-induced hearing loss? *Scandinavian Audiology, 20*(4), 239-244.

Williams W. (2005). Noise exposure levels from personal stereo use. *International Journal of Audiology, 44*(4): 231-236.

Wood, W. S., & Lipscomb, D. M. (1972). Maximum available sound pressure levels from stereo components. *Journal of the Acoustical Society of America, 52,* 484-487.

World Health Organization (WHO). (1995). Community noise. In B. Bergkund & T. Lindvall. (Eds.), *Archives of the Center for Sensory Research 2*(1) pp. 1-195. Stockholm, Sweden: Author

Zobgy, J. (Zogby International). (2006). Survey of teens and adults about the use of personal electronic devices and head phones. *American Speech-Language-Hearing Association.* Retrieved December 31, 2007, from http://www.asha.org/about/news/atitbtot/zogby

6 Uniform Hearing Protection for Musicians

BY PATRICIA A. NIQUETTE

INTRODUCTION

Use of hearing protection by musicians and music industry professionals can dramatically reduce auditory risk; however, standard hearing protectors are generally unacceptable because they provide too much attenuation and they alter the frequency response, making music sound muddy and unclear. Flat-response moderate attenuation earplugs, available in custom and noncustom styles, are the preferred choice for amateur and professional musicians. This chapter discusses the design and rationale of flat attenuation earplugs and provides techniques for fitting and troubleshooting them.

SCOPE OF THE PROBLEM

Decades of data have demonstrated that exposure to loud sound for sustained periods of time can cause noise induced hearing loss, and exposure to loud music is no exception. Chasin (1996) reported that most professional musicians will eventually develop music induced hearing loss, and Royster et al. (1991) found that over half of symphony orchestra musicians had audiometric profiles consistent with noise induced hearing damage. In addition to hearing loss, excessive sound exposures can cause tinnitus, diplacusis (abnormal pitch perception), and hyperacusis, any of which can be debilitating and career threatening to those employed in the music industry. Audio engineers, recording engineers, sound crews, managers, disc jockeys, and music educators, as well as music students, are all exposed to high sound levels and all face a real risk of incurring permanent auditory damage. Typical sound levels that musicians are exposed to can be found in Chapter 1.

KEY POINT

In addition to hearing loss, excessive sound exposures can cause tinnitus, diplacusis, and hyperacusis, any of which can be debilitating and career threatening to those employed in the music industry.

DAMAGE RISK CRITERIA

Damage risk criteria are based on industrial noise, and whereas the music spectrum is quite different, damage risk criteria remain the best guidelines we have at present to estimate auditory risk and the need for hearing protection for music exposures. Two standards exist in the United States: Occupational Safety and Health Administration (OSHA) Occupational Noise Standard (OSHA, 1983) and National Institute for Occupational Safety and Health (NIOSH) Criteria for a Recommended Standard (NIOSH, 1998).

OSHA

When deciding which standard to use, it is important to keep in mind that the differences in these standards have a significant impact on auditory risk. The more liberal OSHA standard provides for a permissible exposure limit (PEL) of 90 dBA for 8 hours per day, 5 days per week, for a working lifetime of 40 years. OSHA uses a 5 dB time-intensity tradeoff; that is, for every 5 dB increase in noise level, the allowable exposure time is reduced by half (Table 6–1). The OSHA standard reflects a compromise between risk reduction and cost implementation for an indus-

trial workforce, and the higher exposure limits result in a greater number of individuals incurring significant hearing loss.

KEY POINT

The OSHA standard uses a 5 dB exchange rate and reflects a compromise between risk reduction and cost implementation for an industrial workforce.

NIOSH

In contrast, the NIOSH criteria have a PEL of 85 dBA for 8 hours per day (5 dB less than the OSHA standard) with a 3 dB time-intensity tradeoff: for every 3 dB increase in noise level, the allowable exposure time is reduced by half. The NIOSH standard is based on scientific data, with an emphasis on hearing loss prevention. The choice of which standard to use impacts the risk of material hearing impairment; with a 40-year (working lifetime) exposure, the OSHA standard results in 25% excess risk for developing a material hearing impairment, whereas the NIOSH criteria result in 8% excess risk (NIOSH, 1998). As reported by Suter (2006), the vast majority of nations around the world use an 8-hour PEL of 85 dB with a 3 dB exchange rate, and in 2007 the Interna-

Table 6–1. Allowable daily exposures (OSHA and NIOSH)

	Noise level dBA							
	85	88	90	92	94	95	97	100
OSHA	16		8	6		4	3	2
NIOSH	8	4			1	3/4	1/2	1/4

Note. Adapted and used with permission from Etymotic Research, Inc.

tional Safety Equipment Association petitioned OSHA to adopt an 85 dBA PEL with a 3 dB exchange rate. It remains to be seen if OSHA will embark on the lengthy process of changing the noise standard.

KEY POINT

The NIOSH standard uses a 3 dB exchange rate and is based on scientific data, with an emphasis on hearing loss prevention.

Noise Dose

Because music levels vary widely, it is difficult to predict an individual's true exposure over time. However, a measure of noise dose (a measure integrating sound levels over time) provides a more accurate estimate of risk. Both the OSHA standard and the NIOSH criteria are based on noise dose, which is expressed as a percentage of the daily maximum permissible exposure. Using the NIOSH criteria, a 100% dose is equivalent to an 85 dBA time-weighted average for 8 hours (or 88 dBA for 4 hours, 91 dBA for 2 hours, and so on). See Table 6–2.

LIMITATIONS OF CONVENTIONAL EARPLUGS

Musicians need protection from excessive sound levels to prevent auditory injury, but they also need to hear, and hear well, while they play. Traditional earplugs are problematic for those in the music industry for three major reasons: unbalanced attenuation (too much high frequency attenuation); too much overall attenuation; and excessive occlusion effect.

Table 6–2. Exposure levels and durations equivalent to a 100% noise dose based on the NIOSH criteria

Level (dBA)	Duration	Dose %
79	24	75
82	16	100
85	8	100
88	4	100
91	2	100
94	1	100
97	30 min	100
100	15 min	100
103	7.5 min	100
106	3.75 min	100

Note. For durations exceeding those shown, the resulting dose is larger; for example, a 91 dB exposure for 4 hours would be twice the daily limit (200% dose); 91 dB for 8 hours would be four times the daily limit (400% dose), and so on.

Unbalanced Attenuation

Inserting an earplug into the ear removes the ear's natural resonant peak, which is approximately 17 dB at 2700 Hz in the average ear. When combined with the earplug's attenuation characteristics, this results in a net treble deficiency of 15 to 20 dB (Killion, 1993), causing music and voices to sound muffled. Most musical instruments have a significant amount of energy above 1000 Hz, with harmonics that are more intense than the fundamental (Chasin, 1996). Earplugs with too much high frequency attenuation destroy the tonal balance, which can result in mishearing or overplaying to compensate for the lack of high frequency sound heard through the earplugs. Overplaying, in turn, can cause other music-related injuries (e.g., wrist strain or injury in drummers).

Too Much Overall Attenuation

Standard hearing protectors often provide too much attenuation for those in the music industry: deeply inserted foam earplugs can provide 30 to 40 dB of sound reduction when far less may be needed to adequately protect hearing. Excessive attenuation can result in mishearing or overplaying, and in this case musicians often forego the use of hearing protection in an effort to hear the music better.

Occlusion Effect

Occlusion effect is an increase in sound pressure level at the eardrum in the occluded ear compared to the open ear for sounds generated by the user (e.g., vocalist, brass, or woodwinds). When a musician sings or blows into the mouthpiece of an instrument, sound is conducted via the jaw to the bone surrounding the inner one third of the ear canal. When earplugs provide a shallow seal (outer two thirds of the ear canal) the result is elevated sound pressure levels behind the earplug, which may put the musician at risk for overexposure.

KEY POINT

Traditional earplugs are problematic for those in the music industry because of unbalanced attenuation, too much overall attenuation, and excessive occlusion effect.

DESIGN AND RATIONALE FOR HIGH FIDELITY EARPLUGS

High fidelity earplugs reproduce sound as it is normally heard, but at a lower intensity, preserving the tonal balance of the music while reducing sound levels at the ear. Musicians Earplugs™ (Killion, DeVilbiss, & Stewart, 1988) were the first and are still the only custom high fidelity earplugs in the world. Musicians Earplugs consist of a deeply-fitted custom earmold combined with a patented attenuator button. As shown in Figure 6–1, the volume of air in the earmold bore acts as an acoustic mass, whereas the diaphragm in the attenuator button acts as an acoustic compliance. The combination of the two produces a resonance at approximately 2700 Hz (as in the average normal ear) resulting in a smooth, flat attenuation across frequency (Killion et al., 1988; Figure 6–2).

Shown another way, Musicians Earplugs preserve the tonal balance of the music, as can be seen in Figure 6–3. The overall level is reduced equally across

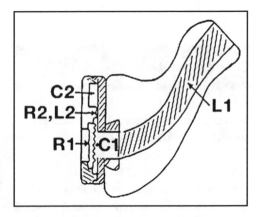

Figure 6–1. Line diagram of ER-15 Musicians Earplug. C = compliance; R = resistance; L = inductance.

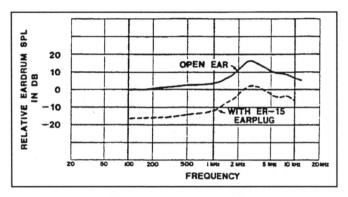

Figure 6–2. Expected eardrum SPL in diffuse (random incidence) sound field with ear open vs. ear occluded with ER-15 earplug. *Note.* From "An Earplug with Uniform 15-dB Attenuation," by M. C. Killion, E. DeVilbiss, & J. Stewart, 1988, *Hear Journal, 41*(4), pp. 14–17. Used with permission.

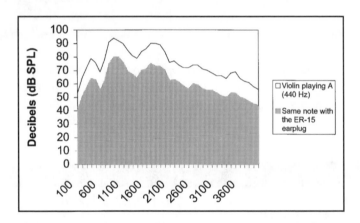

Figure 6–3. Musicians Earplugs preserve the tonal balance of the music. The overall level is reduced equally across the frequency range, thereby maintaining the spectral "shape."

the frequency range, thereby maintaining the "shape" of the music.

KEY POINT

High fidelity earplugs such as the ER-15 reproduce sound as it is normally heard, but at a lower intensity, preserving the tonal balance of the music while reducing sound levels at the ear.

GUIDELINES FOR CHOOSING ATTENUATORS

The interchangeable attenuator buttons are available in three values: 9, 15, and 25 dB, and Musicians Earplugs using these attenuators are referred to as the ER-9, ER-15, and ER-25. The optimal attenuator is the one that provides the minimum amount of attenuation that will reduce sound exposures to a safe level. As mentioned previously, too much attenuation can cause problems for musicians. Fortunately, the actual amount of attenuation needed is often less than one might expect, as Table 6–3 illustrates.

The ER-15 has the flattest frequency response, and is useful for most musical applications, whereas the ER-25 is recommended only for higher sound exposures (e.g., drummers, marching band drumlines, rock musicians, amplified music, and those located in front of the brass section). The ER-9 provides 9 dB of attenuation in the low frequencies and 14 to 15 dB of attenuation in the high frequencies and is often appropriate for solo practice and other situations in which less than 15 dB of protection is needed (e.g., viola players). Musicians often require at least two sets of attenuators (such as ER-15 and ER-25), which are interchangeable depending on the exposure

level; this sometimes means using a different attenuator in each ear. Table 6–4 summarizes these recommendations for various music instrument categories.

Deeply-sealed earplugs are necessary to reduce the occlusion effect; thus, Musicians Earplugs should be long enough to seal deeply in the bony portion of the ear canal (Killion, 2003; Killion et al., 1988). On occasion, a bit of occlusion is desirable (e.g., for vocalists as an aid in self-monitoring), and if needed, this can be achieved with a slightly shorter plug that seals less deeply in the ear canal.

IMPORTANCE OF IMPRESSION TECHNIQUE

Because Musicians Earplugs are a custom product, they're ultimately only as good as the professional who fits them and the

Table 6–3. Limits of permissible exposure based on NIOSH

Level (dBA)	% Dose per Hour	% Dose 8 Hours	Time (Hours) to Reach 100% Dose				
			No EP	ER-9	ER-15	ER-25	ER-20
85	<25 (12.5)	100	8	24	24	24	24
88	25	200	4	24	24	24	24
91	50	400	2	16	24	24	24
94	100	800	1	8	24	24	24
97	200	1600	30 min	4	16	24	24
100	400	3200	15 min	2	8	24	22 (est.)
103	800	6400	7.5 min	1	4	24	14 (est.)
106	1600	12,800	3.8 min	30 min	2	20 (est.)	7 (est.)
109	3200	25,600	1.9 min	15 min	1	10 (est.)	3.5 (est.)

Note. Based on "Criteria for a Recommended Standard: Occupational Noise Exposure—Revised Criteria," by the National Institute for Occupational Safety and Health, 1998, Department of Health and Human Services (NIOSH) Publication No. 98-126.

Table 6–4. Recommended custom earplugs for various musical instrument categories. In some cases there is more than one possible fitting.

Instrument Category	ER-9	ER-15	ER-25	Potential Harmful Sounds
Small strings	✓	✓		Own/other instruments
Large strings	✓	✓		Brass
Woodwinds		✓		Brass, percussion
Brass		✓	✓	Other brass
Flutes		✓		Percussion
Percussion			✓	Own/other percussion
Vocalists	✓	✓		Speakers/monitors
Acoustic guitar	✓	✓		Percussion/speakers
Amplified instruments		✓	✓	Speakers/monitors
Marching bands		✓		Multiple sources
Music teachers		✓		Multiple sources
Recording engineers		✓		Speakers/monitors
Sound crews		✓		Speakers/monitors

earmold lab that makes them. Long impressions (past the second bend of the ear canal) are required so earmold laboratories can make earmolds that seal in the bony portion of the ear canal. Musicians may require extra reassurance while long impressions are taken. Whenever possible, musicians should play their instrument while the impressions are curing so that all normal mouth, jaw, and body movements (which affect the shape of the ear canal) are accounted for in the finished impressions (Santucci, personal communication, February 16, 2007). Impressions should have no gaps, and should extend past the second bend of the ear canal. Even experienced clinicians redo impressions, because properly fitting Musicians Earplugs cannot be made from inadequate impressions. Seal issues can often be resolved by taking impres-

sions using a high viscosity silicone (Pirzanski, 2006). The musician should hold her mouth open while the silicone is injected, and then make normal movements (as in playing the instrument) while the impression is curing.

EARMOLD CONSTRUCTION

The sole manufacturer of attenuators for Musicians Earplugs is Etymotic Research, Inc. Earmold laboratories are held to rigorous standards of construction, so that earplugs made by any lab in the world should provide the same flat attenuation in the ear. Etymotic Research and its European affiliate conduct regular site visits to ensure uniform manufacturing practices. Labs use the same fundamental principles to determine sound bore dimensions and canal length, which produce flat attenuation when the buttons are attached to the custom earmolds. This is accomplished in part by measuring the correct volume of air in the finished mold with an acoustic mass meter. Certification is awarded to a lab when all criteria are met.

ORDERING OPTIONS

Earmolds for Musicians Earplugs are available in silicone or vinyl, with silicone having the advantage of significantly less shrinkage over time (Dillon, 2001). Typically one set of attenuator buttons is supplied with the earmolds, but additional attenuators can be ordered from the earmold lab at the time of the original order or at a later date. Attenuator buttons are available in clear, beige, red, or blue, and can be partially countersunk or completely countersunk into the earmolds (Figure 6–4).

FITTING MUSICIANS EARPLUGS

Musicians Earplugs should be fitted as part of a hearing loss prevention program that includes comprehensive baseline audio-logical testing and ongoing monitoring. Earplugs reduce sound levels at the ear only if a seal is achieved and they are worn consistently. Audiological monitoring provides the evidence needed to determine if the hearing loss prevention program is working. Musicians Earplugs require a professional fitting and orientation that includes verification of earmold fit and instruction on use and care of the earplugs. Earplugs should not cause discomfort or soreness, although a modified wearing schedule may be necessary at first for plugs that seal deeply. As with most earmolds, Musicians Earplugs can be washed with mild soap and water (after removing attenuator buttons). Vinyl molds will eventually shrink and harden over time, whereas silicone molds remain more stable (Dillon, 2001).

VERIFICATION OF PERFORMANCE

The attenuation of Musicians Earplugs can be measured using standard real-ear measurement protocols (measuring insertion loss rather than insertion gain). Real-ear measures can also be used to assess the degree of occlusion effect and the results of any corrective actions. Techniques for these measures are described by Chasin (1996, 1998), Revit (1992,

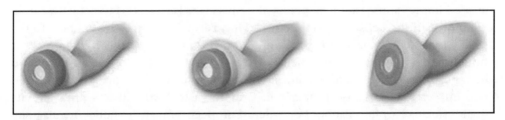

Figure 6–4. Custom Musicians Earplugs with attenuators placed. Standard, partially countersunk, and countersunk.

2000), and Mueller et al. (1992). The most common fitting issue encountered is reduced low frequency attenuation (unbalanced attenuation) caused by a leak in the earmold fit. When this occurs, the earmolds should be remade from new impressions. An occlusion effect of 20 dB is significant and should also be addressed by having the earmolds remade. Fit problems can often be successfully addressed by using a high viscosity silicone impression material and an open-jaw impression technique (Pirzanski, 2006). Every ear is unique and in some cases the geometry of the user's ear canals will impact the response of the finished product. Narrow ear canals can be particularly problematic; if the earmolds are long enough to seal in the bony portion of the ear canal, the bore diameter may not be wide enough to provide the high frequency boost needed to overcome insertion loss. Shortening the earmolds allows for a wider bore and better high frequency response but may increase the occlusion effect (which may not be an issue if the musician isn't a vocalist or horn player). The needs of each user must be taken into account in this situation.

NON-CUSTOM EARPLUGS FOR MUSICIANS

Shortly after the introduction of Musicians Earplugs, Etymotic Research and Aearo Corporation jointly developed and patented the ER-20™, a low cost, ready-fit, high fidelity earplug. The ER-20s use a tuned resonator and acoustic resistor (Figure 6–5) to provide an almost-flat 20 dB of sound reduction across frequency.

As with custom Musicians Earplugs, the optimal response with ER-20s (flat

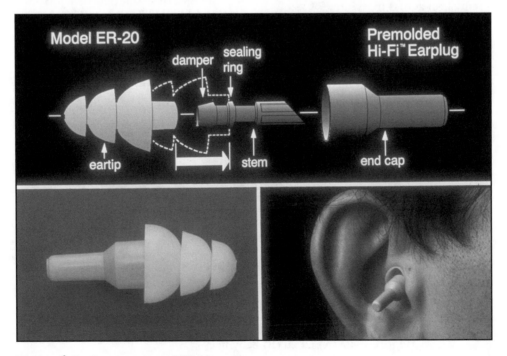

Figure 6–5. Construction of ER-20 earplug.

attenuation with little occlusion effect) is achieved when the earplugs seal deeply in the ear canals. Whereas the ER-20s fit most average size ears, they're too large for some adult ears and many children's ears. The ER-20 earplug shown in Figure 6–6a seals the ear, although not deeply. More importantly, the user reported it was uncomfortable and thus unlikely to be worn consistently. In 2006, Etymotic Research released BabyBlues™ earplugs, which provide the same 20 dB of flat attenuation as the ER-20s but have smaller eartips to fit smaller-than-average-size ear canals. The BabyBlues earplug shown in Figure 6–6b provides a deeper seal, and the same user reported it was comfortable for long periods of time.

KEY POINT

The noncustom ER-20s use a tuned resonator and acoustic resistor to provide an almost-flat 20 dB of sound reduction across frequency.

The ER-20s and BabyBlues provide a high fidelity, low cost option so anyone can benefit from flat attenuation hearing protection. These earplugs are used by thousands of music educators and students in the United States. The most successful programs require the use of hearing protection for students exposed to damaging sound levels in school-based and school-sponsored activities (Palmer, 2007). These earplugs are also useful as a backup for anyone who uses custom Musicians Earplugs.

NOISE REDUCTION RATING (NRR)

The U.S. EPA requires manufacturers to print a noise reduction rating (NRR) on all noncustom earplugs. The required formula used to determine NRR includes an adjustment for individual variability and for those persons who do not wear ear protection as instructed. Many investigators have found no consistent rank order correlation between the real-world NRRs and labeled NRRs (Berger, 1999). NRR is computed from laboratory data that are not representative of the values attained in the real world by actual users. The NRR for the ER-20s is 12 dB, but clinical measurements of properly inserted ER-20s

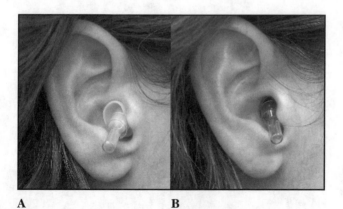

A   B

Figure 6–6. (A) ER-20 (B) BabyBlues.

indicate they provide almost equal sound reduction (20 dB) at all frequencies (E-A-RCAL, 1992).

SUMMARY

Musicians and music industry professionals are at significant risk of developing permanent auditory damage from high sound levels. Suggested exposure limits in the United States are based on two standards: Occupational Safety and Health Administration (OSHA) Occupational Noise Standard (OSHA, 1983) and National Institute for Occupational Safety and Health (NIOSH) Criteria for a Recommended Standard (NIOSH, 1998). The OSHA standard uses a 5 dB exchange rate that predicts less potential damage for a given exposure than does the NIOSH standard, which uses the 3 dB exchange rate. The 3 dB exchange rate is based on solid scientific studies. Both the OSHA and the NIOSH standards are based on noise dose, which is expressed as a percentage of the daily maximum permissible exposure.

Traditional earplugs are problematic for those in the music industry because of unbalanced attenuation, too much overall attenuation, and excessive occlusion effect. Custom Musician Earplugs (ER-9, ER-15, and ER-25) provide uniform attenuation, and when used properly minimize the risk for future hearing loss while still allowing the musician to be able to hear and monitor music. Noncustom versions (ER-20 and BabyBlues) provide a low cost, ready-fit option appropriate for all music enthusiasts.

Acknowledgment. Dr. Niquette is an audiologist at Etymotic Research, Inc.

REFERENCES

Berger, E. H. (1993). *The naked truth about NRRs (EARLog 20)*. Indianapolis, IN: E-A-R Hearing Protection Products.

Berger, E. H. (1999). So, how do you want your NRRs: Realistic or sunny-side-up? *Hearing Review*, 6(9), 68–72.

Chasin, M. (1996). *Musicians and the prevention of hearing loss*. San Diego, CA: Singular.

Chasin, M. (1998). Assessing musicians. Audio-Scan App Note. Dorchester, Ontario: Etymonic Design, Inc. Retrieved December 18, 2007, from http://www.audioscan.com/resources/appnotes/AppNote_98-05.pdf

Dillon, H. (2001). Hearing aid earmolds, earshells and coupling systems. *Hearing Aids*. New York: Thieme.

E-A-RCAL. (1992). Acoustical laboratory test report per ANSI S.3.19-1974. Indianapolis, IN: Kieper RW and Berger EH

Killion, M. C. (1988). The hollow voice occlusion effect. Hearing aid fitting: Theoretical and practical views. In J. H. Jensen (Ed.), *13th Danavox Symposium* (pp. 231–241). Copenhagen, Denmark: Stougaard Jensen.

Killion, M. C. (1993). The parvum bonum, plus melius fallacy in earplug selection. Recent developments in hearing instrument technology. In J. Beilin & G. R. Jensen (Eds.), *15th Danavox Symposium* (pp. 415–433). Copenhagen, Denmark: Stougaard Jensen.

Killion, M. C. (2003). Earmold acoustics. *Seminars in Hearing*, 24(4), 299–312.

Killion, M. C., DeVilbiss, E., & Stewart, J. (1988). An earplug with uniform 15-dB attenuation. *Hearing Journal*, 41(4), 14–17.

Mueller, H. G., Hawkins, D. B., & Northern, J. L. (1992). *Probe microphone measurements*. San Diego, CA: Singular.

National Institute for Occupational Safety and Health. (1998). *Criteria for a recommended standard: Occupational noise exposure—Revised criteria*. U.S. Department of Health and Human Services (NIOSH) Publication No. 98-126.

Occupational Safety and Health Administration. (1983). Department of Labor Occupational Noise Exposure Standard, 29 CFR 1910.95.

Palmer, C. V. (2007). Hearing protection for young musicians. *Spectrum, 24*(3), 1, 8–9.

Pirzanski, C. (2006). Earmolds and hearing aid shells: A tutorial. Part 2: Impression-taking techniques that result in fewer remakes. *Hearing Review, 13*(5), 39–46.

Revit, L. J. (1992). Two techniques for dealing with the occlusion effect. *Hearing Instruments, 43*(12), 16–18.

Revit, L. J. (2000). Real-ear measures. In M. Valente, H, Hosford-Dunn, & R. J. Roeser (Eds.), *Audiology Treatment* (pp 114–115.). New York: Thieme.

Royster, J. D., Royster, L. H., & Killion, M. C. (1991). Sound exposures and hearing thresholds of symphony orchestra musicians. *Journal of the Acoustical Society of America, 89*(6), 2793–2803.

Suter, A. H. (2006). *Position paper on regulation of occupational noise exposure.* Reprinted in: *JobHealth Highlights, 25*(5, 8). Retrieved December 18, 2007, from http://hearinglossprevention.org

7 Personal In-the-Ear Monitoring: The Audiologist's Role

BY MICHAEL SANTUCCI

During live performances, musicians need to hear themselves on stage over a myriad of competing sound sources. The PA system, crowd noise, and high on-stage volume levels from other band members trying to hear themselves all add to the difficulty in hearing one's own instrument or voice during a live performance. As a result, escalating on-stage sound levels have become a constant problem for musicians, their sound engineers, and crew, as well as fans from all genres of music (Morlet, Santucci, & Morlet, 2007).

In-the-ear monitors (IEM), also called personal monitors, are designed to eliminate the need for floor-mounted loudspeakers. IEM systems have come a long way in terms of sound quality and comfort since their inception in the late 1980s.

This chapter will compare and contrast traditional on-stage monitor speakers with today's IEM systems and, most importantly, discuss the role of the audiologist in helping select the appropriate earpiece and guiding the musician in safe use.

TRADITIONAL ON-STAGE MONITORING: BRIEF DESCRIPTION

Because the audio from the main public address system is aimed out at the audience, the sound is delayed before it reflects back to the stage, making it extremely difficult for musicians to play in time with each other. The solution has been to place additional loudspeakers on stage and turn them around to face the artists. These highly directional speakers, often called *wedges* owing to their shape, are typically placed on the stage in front of the musician. Additional speakers (called *side-fills*) are often added to both sides of the stage to provide even more sound reinforcement for the performers. In essence, this creates a second, separate sound system for the musicians, called the *monitor system*.

Concerts of this magnitude require two sound engineers. The front of house (FOH) engineer mixes the main public address sound system for the audience, usually working from a sonically strategic position near the center and toward the rear of the main floor. By contrast, the monitor engineer (ME) works out of sight from the side of the stage, creating separate mixes for each musician and routing those mixes to the wedges at their performing positions. This allows each musician to hear an individually tailored mix.

These loudspeaker monitor systems present a variety of problems for the performers, the audience, and the engineers. The proximity of the wedges to the microphones increases the possibility of feedback. At the same time, the tendency among the performers is to request more volume in their monitors to hear themselves over the competing sound sources (the FOH system, drum kits, guitar amps, and nearby wedges). This typically results in needlessly intense sound levels on stage. Thus, the monitor engineer faces a constant balancing act—trying to keep the musicians happy while still preventing acoustic feedback from the wedges. At the same time, the FOH engineer has no choice but to increase the volume of the house speakers to override the on-stage monitor system that is now spilling out into the audience, interfering with the quality of the main FOH mix. The audience in turn suffers through excessive sound levels and compromises in the sound quality of the FOH mix.

KEY POINT

When working with musicians, it's important to remember that their primary focus is the performance, and for some, hearing protection may be secondary.

PERSONAL MONITORING

In response to this situation, the first in-ear monitoring systems were developed in the late 1980s. In much the way that the Sony Walkman replaced "boom box" portable stereos, IEMs were designed to move the musician's on-stage listening experience directly into the ears. This approach eliminates the competition between sound sources inherent in a wedge system, allowing musicians to hear themselves more precisely while eliminating the biggest single source of feedback on stage.

An IEM system consists of a belt-pack amplifier that is either hard-wired or wireless, and a set of earphones with tiny loudspeakers. Wireless systems use a UHF radio link to send the mix to the performer, who is now always "in the sweet spot"—hearing the same mix everywhere on stage. Stationary performers, such as drummers and keyboard players, typically use hard-wired systems.

Originally little more than consumer earbuds, today's earphones are sophisticated audio devices, designed to create isolation from competing sound sources while presenting a high fidelity signal. Various manufacturers offer either universal-fit or custom-fit designs. Because ear impressions are required for custom molds, the services of an audiologist are also required.

For performers, an IEM system offers numerous benefits over traditional stage wedges. By presenting the mix directly in the ear, musicians gain improved pitch perception and musical timing. And with the isolation from ambient sound provided by the earphones, it also becomes possible to monitor more accurately at lower volume levels. Finally, the stage show itself can be improved, as performers no longer need to stand in front of their wedges in order to hear accurately.

MEs benefit by gaining the ability to present a consistent monitor mix, night after night, whatever the conditions in the venue. Volume levels are controlled by the musicians' body-packs, leaving the ME free to concentrate on the quality of the mixes themselves. And by eliminating monitor wedges from the stage, the chances for feedback are greatly reduced. For the same reason, FOH engineers can create a more cohesive, high fidelity mix and can present it at safer levels. Ultimately, even the audience benefits.

Because the objective of on-stage monitor systems is to allow the performers to hear themselves, and given the above-mentioned limitations of wedges, it is no surprise that the personal monitoring concept has been embraced throughout the live sound industry and is being used increasingly even in smaller venues.

PERSONAL MONITOR EARPHONES

As the demand for this technology becomes more prevalent, audiologists may see an increasing number of musicians requesting "ear impressions" for custom-molded IEMs. Because concert sound reinforcement strategies are foreign to most of us, it is critical for the audiologist to learn how to provide quality service to this new client base.

Before one can provide guidance on selection and safe use of earphones for IEM systems, it's important to have a basic understanding of earpiece technology. Like hearing aids, an important aspect to successful personal monitoring is the quality and fit of the earpieces. IEM earphones come in three types: consumer-style earbuds, universal-fit earphones, and custom-molded earphones.

The goal is to provide a full bandwidth stereo mix to the performer on stage, while acoustically blocking out the competing sound sources. Good earphone designs allow the performer to hear more detail than is possible with floor monitors, allowing reduced sound levels at the ear. Earbud type earphones such as those used with portable MP3 players are not favored for on-stage applications, as their "on ear" design does not offer the degree of isolation required. For this reason, IEM designs dominate the marketplace.

Most IEM systems are sold with a pair of universal-fit earphones along with the wireless or hard-wired audio system, offering the musician immediate usability. These earphones come with a variety of generic tip couplers, ranging from foam cylinders to plastic or silicone mushroom caps and triple flanged shapes, providing the user with options for the best comfort and isolation from ambient sound. Some models can be upgraded with a custom sleeve mold to provide more comfort and isolation, which is preferred for active performers or those with small or sharply bending ear canals. These custom attachments are made of soft materials, much like a power behind-the-ear (BTE) mold (Figure 7–1 and 7–2).

The best fit, comfort, and sound quality come from custom-molded earpieces, used by virtually all performers who can afford them. Resembling in-the-ear hearing aids, the custom earphone completely encases microspeakers that are positioned within each unique mold in a way that is more cosmetic and comfortable than universal-fit earphones. These custom

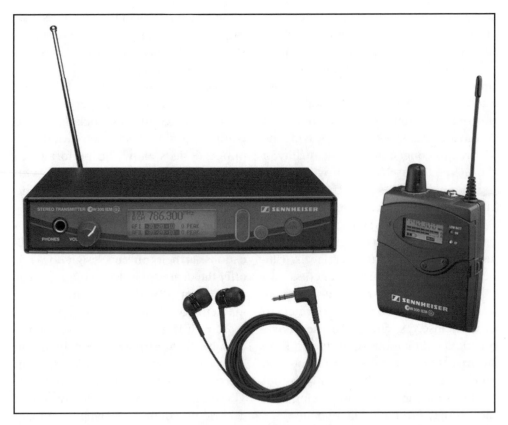

Figure 7–1. Photo of an in-ear monitor (IEM) system showing the transmitter and wireless receiver worn by the musician. *Note.* Courtesy of Sennheiser. Used with permission.

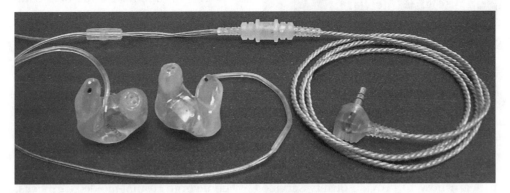

Figure 7–2. Photo of of a custom made in-ear monitor (IEM). *Note.* Courtesy of Sesaphonics. Used with permission.

personal monitors come in a variety of materials including soft (silicone), hard (acrylic), and hard acrylic with soft acrylic canal. Because artists typically make exaggerated facial movements while performing, soft materials seem to provide the best isolation and comfort during extended use.

The microspeakers used are categorized as either dynamic or balanced armature type. Dynamic diaphragms (such as those found in typical MP3 type earbuds) are designed for the open ear canal and need air vents on the outside of the casing to allow full movement of the diaphragm. Consequently, custom monitors with dynamic type speakers offer little or no isolation because of the venting needed for maximized sound quality. Balanced armature speakers are the same type of speaker found in hearing aid technology. However, because musicians require full bandwidth reproduction, special hybrid drivers and, more recently, active speaker technology, are employed. These transducers may be offered as a wide-band single driver or in combinations of two or three, to satisfy the musician's desire for a fuller bass response. Musicians should be warned that excessive levels can be damaging and that an audiologist be sought out to verify the output levels. Balanced armature designs are more widely available than dynamics because of their improved sound quality, and they isolate the ear from ambient sound, thereby enhancing the signal- (monitor mix) to-noise (competing sound sources; S/N) ratio in the ear canal. It would be tempting to conclude that the better the S/N ratio, the lower the sound level needed to hear accurately. However, this is only typically the case after counseling regarding proper use is provided. In short, custom-fit designs using soft materials provide the greatest amount of isolation, which in turn improves the sound quality delivered from balanced armature transducers, thereby offering the possibility that the user can hear accurately at safer levels.

Ironically (or perhaps inevitably), isolation also creates a new problem for the musician. Performers complain of feeling detached from the audience, and fellow band members often remove one earpiece in order to "feel the room again" or to communicate with band mates or the audience between songs. Inventive monitor engineers have maximized monitor mixes using advanced audio tools, often "miking" the audience to include the room sound in the monitor mix, replicating what one would hear without something occluding the ear. Although these techniques have partially remedied musician complaints associated with isolating monitors, they do not allow the musician to use the reflective properties of the head and pinna needed for localization. This is typically the main objection to going in-ear.

To address this obstacle several IEM manufacturers have developed in situ microphones that work in conjunction with the monitor system. These tiny, hybrid microphones, designed to take high SPL peaks without overloading, are embedded in the earpieces and can be equalized to the average response of an open ear canal. The ambient sound is now completely natural while directionality cues are retained. The sound from these ambient microphones is sent to a body-pack, where an active circuit combines the audio from the microphones with the input from the monitor system at the desired relative levels, producing a full mix of music and local ambient sound at the ear. As a result, the artist can speak with band mates and hear the audience response during a performance while retaining the benefits of isolation.

THE ROLE OF THE AUDIOLOGIST

When working with musicians, it's important to remember that their primary focus is the performance; all other considerations are secondary. The sound reinforcement gear is only there to help make the show a success. In the case of the monitor system, the expectation is that it enhances the performance by providing the artists with the ability to accurately hear what they are playing. For some musicians, hearing protection is a secondary consideration, although for others it is paramount.

Obviously, musicians are different from the typical audiology client. For this reason, it is imperative that the audiologist take the lead in teaching how to use IEMs safely. Unlike earplugs, personal monitors are not safety devices by design. In fact, IEM systems are miniature sound systems capable of producing very high sound levels.

KEY POINT

Despite their ability to deliver high quality audio while isolating the ear, for some musicians, IEM systems may not typically be used in a way that affords optimal hearing protection.

Given this concern, how does one direct the musician to safe use, and more importantly, how does the musician decide what is a safe level to monitor? One method is to measure the sound levels from an IEM while in use during a sound check or rehearsals, through probe tube microphone equipment. This portable and clinically available tool can take measurements at the eardrum with the earphone in place. Correction factors need to be used to compensate for the ear canal resonance and for conversion into an A-weighted format. From these readings, musicians can be directed to safe levels using time-weighted averages. More information on potentially damaging levels can be found in Chapter 6.

SAFE USE OF PERSONAL MONITORS

It should be noted that club musicians play an average of 3 hours a night for as many nights per week as possible. Consequently, the safe limits must be lowered in accordance with time of exposure. Much probe tube microphone equipment is not portable or designed for A-weighted measurements, so very few musicians have ever experienced it. As a consequence, most musicians are left to make the judgment of what is too loud on their own.

A study of users of personal monitors suggests that musicians tend to match the levels they were accustomed to while using floor monitors (Federman & Ricketts, 2008). In this study a group of 15 professional musicians were asked to do two things in random order in the same test session: They were asked to (a) turn the stage volume to the level at which they typically perform (preferred listening level, or PLL), and (b) reduce the volume and find the lowest level at which they would still be able to play (minimal acceptable listening level, or MALL). The purpose of the study was to determine the PLL and MALL differences between floor monitors and personal monitors.

The results revealed that all 15 musicians consistently turned their PLL to the same level each day—within 1 dB. In another set of sessions, the subjects were asked to perform the same tasks while using personal monitors. Not surprisingly, subjects demonstrated the same consistency. In addition, PLLs while using IEMs were just as high as they were for the open ear measurements—again, to within less than 1 dB—despite the superior isolation and fidelity of the systems. In other words, the PLL for all 15 musicians was the same whether or not the IEMs were employed.

The good news from a hearing conservation viewpoint is that when using personal monitors, the MALL was 6 dB lower than the PLL. Conversely, the difference between PLL and MALL was only 1 dB when using traditional floor monitors. This suggests that sound levels can be reduced by using IEMs in place of floor wedges, but only with the proper recommendations of an audiologist. More research is still required as we do not know whether floor monitor wedges with hearing protection are better or worse than IEMs at the MALL.

KEY POINT

Sound levels can be reduced by using personal monitors in place of floor wedges, but only with the proper use.

SOME HELPFUL TIPS

Following are some helpful tips to offer the musician client:

1. Test and retest hearing. Although this is not mandatory (as it is in many industries), baseline testing is still the foundation of any successful hearing conservation effort, and musicians should be strongly encouraged to participate. Annual checkups should be the norm. Identifying small changes in a short time sure beats finding larger ones after a few years of use.

2. Recommend isolating custom earphones. The softer the material, the greater degree of isolation with excessive jaw movements.

3. Wear both earpieces—always! Removing one monitor causes the listener to increase the volume in the occluded ear to compensate for the loss of binaural summation. At the same time, the open, unprotected ear is exposed to loud ambient sound levels. Furthermore, volume entering through the open ear can contribute to central masking, again resulting in the musician turning up the single monitor in order to perceive the same volume as when both monitors are used. Recommend using stationary ambient (audience) microphones or earpieces with integrated microphones as a safe method for resolving problems associated with isolation. In some cases proper use of hearing protection may improve the situation.

4. Use peak limiters or compressors. Most personal monitor systems include a peak limiter in the amplifier/receiver belt pack. Some sound engineers prefer to use onboard limiters. Both methods help protect the user from loud, unexpected bursts of sound and are an important link of the preservation chain. Of course, this does not prevent the performer from turning the volume to unsafe levels.

5. Avoid venting the monitor. Venting the earphone (in an effort to regain lost ambient sound) not only results in a reduction of bass response with armature type transducers, but also allows stage volume to bleed into the ear uncontrollably, eliminating the benefits of isolation.

6. Be aware of warning signs such as tinnitus and temporary threshold

shift after a performance, and reduce volume levels and exposure times accordingly.

SUMMARY

The inability of musicians to hear themselves clearly on stage, even in small venues and clubs, causes them to turn their monitor system and on-stage amplifiers to unsafe levels in an effort to hear over competing sound sources, including other band members, the public address loudspeakers, and crowd noise. IEMs or personal monitors can enhance the on-stage listening experience.

Despite their ability to deliver high quality audio while isolating the ear, IEM systems are not typically being used in a way that affords hearing protection. However, with proper instruction (including counseling, education, and verification with real-ear measurement tools), they have great potential to protect the hearing of at-risk musicians.

Baseline and regular follow-up audiometric testing can track possible changes in hearing from improper IEM use. This is particularly important if the tools to measure IEM output levels in situ are not available. Skilled advice on the importance of using earpieces, isolating molds, and peak limiters or compressors can contribute to preserving the valuable hearing of this growing client base, thus prolonging the careers of these performers, who give us so much through their music.

Acknowledgment. Michael Santucci is the president of Sensaphonics—a manufacturer of IEMs.

REFERENCES

Federman, J., & Ricketts, T. (2008). Preferred and minimum acceptable listening levels for musicians while using floor and in-ear monitors. *Journal of Speech Language Hearing Research, 51*(1), 147–160.

Morlet, S., Santucci, M., & Morlet, T. (2007). *Musicians and hearing loss: Comparison to a non noise exposed population incidence and risk factors.* Paper presented at American Academy of Audiology Conference, Denver, CO.

8 Room and Stage Acoustics for Optimal Listening and Playing

BY WILLIAM J. GASTMEIER

Typically, the focus of the design of a performance arts facility is to achieve a superior acoustical experience for the audience. Considerations of sound propagation, sound quality, reverberation, even audience coverage, low background noise, sufficient direct sound, and sufficient early reflected energy seem to take precedence over the needs of the musician.

In this chapter, we deal with acoustical design aspects of performance and rehearsal spaces intended to enhance the performing artists' experience as well as that of the audience. These are professional workplaces that should as much as possible be designed with health and safety considerations in mind. Musicians need to work in acoustically comfortable environments that enhance their performance, allow them to clearly hear themselves and each other, play as a cohesive unit, and be heard by the audience without undue strain and avoiding excessive levels of sound to minimize the risk of hearing damage.

CONCERT HALLS AND AUDITORIUMS

The best workplace of all is a well-designed performance hall. Since the time of Wallace Sabine, who was considered to be the father of modern architectural acoustics, much research has been devoted to determining those factors that contribute to "good acoustics" in concert halls. Dr. Leo Beranek has recently completed an extensive review of 100 music halls around the world (Beranek, 2004) and has distilled through interview and measurement that most musicians and music lovers can agree that, to provide an optimum listening experience, a hall must be so quiet that very soft (*pp*) passages are audible and sufficiently reverberant to carry crescendos to dramatic very loud (*ff*) climaxes, provide sufficient clarity to support rapidly moving violin passages, provide a spaciousness that increases the apparent size of the instruments, provide a pleasant texture to the music, empart sufficient bass power to the orchestra to solidly support it, and be free of echoes or source shifts. Similar work was conducted in the former Soviet Union (Makrinenko, 1994).

These researchers and many others have developed an extensive terminology and a number of quantitative measures in this regard. These parameters (used in the text in italics) can be generally collected into the four essential categories discussed below, in the context of hearing health and its implications to musicians.

These four categories are (a) an adequately intense performance sound level and low background sound levels, (b) sufficient early sound reflections, (c) sound that is evenly distributed throughout the hall, and (d) reverberation characteristics that are appropriate for the music being played. It is the proper balance of all these parameters to which designers strive, not just for the benefit of the listeners, but also for the musicians and performers.

ADEQUATELY INTENSE PERFORMANCE SOUND LEVEL AND LOW LEVELS OF BACKGROUND SOUND

Early outdoor Greek and Roman amphitheaters are known to have good acoustics for drama and instrumental recitals by small groups, even though they had relatively low levels of performance sound at significant distance from the performer (Campbell & Greated, 1987). This is because sound naturally decreases with distance. Elevating the performers on a stage to face the audience optimized

vocal intelligibility. Raked seating was used to provide good sight lines and minimize additional audience attenuation (Egan, 1988). The orchestra was placed on a flat reflective surface and overhangs or shells were used to reflect additional sound to the audience. Background sound levels were considerably lower than exist in modern day.

When performance moved indoors, the opportunity became available to increase the performance sound levels through the use of reflections from walls and ceilings. Sufficient *Loudness* or *Strength of Sound* is very important to some musical experience, as is evidenced by the popularity of fortissimo passages at the close of a piece. Large audiences, large distances from the stage, and large physical volumes tend to decrease loudness, so true fortissimo is difficult or impossible to achieve in very large halls. Conversely, loudness is increased if areas of carpet, heavily upholstered seating, and absorptive treatments are minimized, and some activities can be overwhelming in small halls. Consider a full brass band in a small high school gymnatorium!

In large proscenium style theaters, stage shells have been developed to enhance the propagation of sound from the stage house into the audience, with the added benefit of enhancing the musicians' ability to hear one another without playing excessively loudly. Hanging reflective panels, sometimes called clouds or baffles, are used to reflect additional sound energy to the seating areas. These panels must be large and dense (at least 20 kg per square meter) to reflect low frequency sound and increase the *Warmth*, *Bass* (low frequency) *Ratio*, and *Bass Strength*. Thin, relatively lightweight wall or stage constructions such as drywall or wood panels (less than 1 inch thick) actually absorb significant bass energy, and their use is discouraged in performance spaces. Maintaining high values of these parameters allows the projection of a warm sound to the audience without overplaying.

To allow the audience to experience the full dynamic range of a musical performance, the background sound levels must be extremely low. This also allows musicians to play at a comfortable level and still be heard. The theater building is designed to eliminate all outdoor sources of sound, sometimes constructing rooms within rooms for very high levels of acoustical isolation. The introduction of air conditioning systems solved an age-old concern of variable acoustics with temperature and humidity, but introduced a new source of noise. Modern venues are equipped with ultra-quiet low velocity HVAC systems, and the background sound levels can be designed and measured to confirm the results. Sound levels as low as NCB-15 (20 dBA) (Table 8–1) are required for critical spaces, almost as

quiet as the threshold of hearing! A good description of the NCB rating system is given in Beranek (1988).

Russell Johnson, one of the world's greatest concert hall designers, was quoted in his recent obituary: "You have to work very carefully to get the silence right. The acoustician builds his signature on that silence."

EARLY FIRST SOUND REFLECTIONS

The human ear has an innate ability to prefer the early sound arriving from a source (direct sound plus first reflections) and analyzes it in order to gain useful information concerning the source. The ear tends to disregard the later arriving sound that contains higher order reflections or reflections from distant surfaces, which merge into the reverberation pattern of the room. These multiple sound reflections are illustrated in Figures 8–1a and 8–1b.

Table 8–1. Desired background sound levels, NCB Rating System (not including occupant noise)

Venue Type	Background Sound, NCB and (dBA)
Concert halls, opera halls, and recital halls for excellent listening conditions	10 to 15 (18 to 23)
Large auditoriums, large drama theaters, and large churches for very good listening conditions	Not to exceed 20 (28)
Small auditoriums, small churches, and large conference rooms	Not to exceed 30 (38)
Private or semiprivate offices and small conference rooms	30 to 40 (38 to 48)

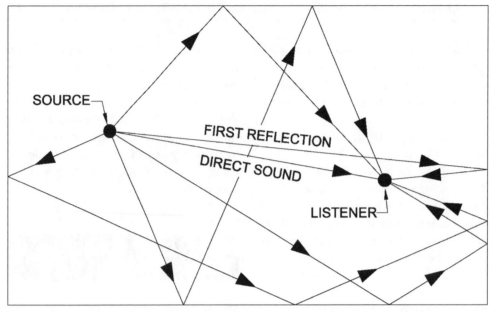

A

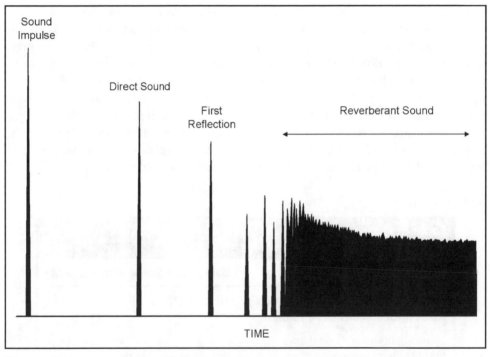

B

Figure 8–1. (**A**) Multiple reflections from the walls of a room of a single impulse produced by a sound source. *Note.* From *The Acoustical Foundations of Music* (p. 145), by J. Backus, 1977, New York: W. W. Norton & Company, Inc. Copyright 1977 by W. W. Norton & Company, Inc. Used with permission. (**B**) Multiple reflections of a sound impulse as heard by a listener. *Note.* From *The Acoustical Foundations of Music* (p. 145), by J. Backus, 1977, New York: W. W. Norton & Company, Inc. Copyright 1977 by W. W. Norton & Company, Inc. Used with permission.

The early work of Beranek (1962), Ando and Gottlob (1979), and others has indicated that if the first reflection arrives less than 20 to 22 ms after the initial direct sound, the *Initial Time Delay Gap*, there is a feeling of *Intimacy*. For near rectangular halls, it can be simply calculated from the architectural drawings, and accurately determined through echograms conducted on scale models or computer modeling. An *Echo* is perceived if a strong reflection arrives more than 80 ms after the direct sound, and Beranek's later work (2004) indicates that *Texture* of the sound is improved if there are a large number of relatively equally spaced reflections before that time.

KEY POINT

A well-designed performance space with adequately sufficient early sound reflections, even sound distribution, and appropriate reverberation greatly benefits the performers as well as the listeners.

Lateral reflections are also quite important. The ratio of lateral to vertical reflections, known as the *Lateral Fraction* (LF), correlates well with the *Apparent Source Width*. This is because our ears are situated in the horizontal plane and we use interaural cues to determine the location and width of sources. Another related parameter, the *Binaural Quality Index*, is one of the most effective indicators of the acoustical quality of concert halls (Beranek, 2004). Both measure the amounts of early arriving (less than 80 ms) laterally reflected sound energy.

However, because sound traverses a distance of approximately 7 m in 20 ms, listeners who sit further than 7 m from

a wall would not feel as intimate as those who sit nearer the walls. This issue does come up in larger theaters, although much of the music performed in larger halls is understandably of a less intimate nature (symphonic works, for example) than that performed in a smaller hall (chamber music or opera). In some instances, variable elements such as moveable stage shell elements, canopies, absorptive banners or curtains, and even loge seating can be introduced to optimize early reflections and provide additional reverberation control if required.

Clearly, it is important for a musician to maintain well-balanced hearing in both ears to benefit from these interaural cues in terms of hearing other musicians and the sound of the orchestra as a whole in the hall.

EVENLY DISTRIBUTED SOUND

A number of acoustical phenomena, known as *Acoustic Defects*, can occur in spaces to interfere with the even distribution of sound around the audience area. In smaller rooms, large parallel surfaces can be an acoustic defect as they can produce *Standing Waves*, through constructive and destructive interference of the incident and reflected waves. Another related defect is *Flutter Echo*, a series of closely spaced echoes that occur when an initial impulse passes repeatedly by the listener. In fact, the simple presence of a large, flat surface can cause such more minor defects such as *Acoustical Glare* and *Source Shift*. Finally, some locations in a performance hall can be significantly louder or quieter than others that are just a little distance away due to improperly oriented reflective surfaces or the presence of *Sound Focusing* from convex reflective surfaces.

These defects can be identified during the initial design and corrected through the application of absorptive or diffusing treatments, or reorienting surfaces or clouds, as discussed below. The extensive use of absorptive treatments such as curtains with pleats to correct such deficiencies can itself pose a problem in terms of destroying the natural reverberation and should be used judiciously as discussed in further sections.

> ### KEY POINT
>
> Acoustic defects such as standing waves, sound focusing, flutter echoes, acoustic glare, and source shift should be avoided.

Computer aided design techniques such as ray tracing, acoustical modeling, and auralization allow the virtual construction of a facility, and have resulted in better designs being put into practice and avoided costly embarrassments. The orientation of reflective surfaces can be fine tuned through the application of geometric or ray acoustics, where the analogy for high frequency (treble) sound is drawn with optics (light and mirrors). Figure 8–2a illustrates the law of reflection, which states that the angle of reflection is equal to the angle of incidence. (Figure 8–2b shows how for large, smooth surfaces, the tilt of each surface can be selected to provide even coverage of the seating areas, both in the horizontal and the vertical planes.)

Scale modeling can be utilized in the design of a concert hall by using a spark generator located on the stage of the model. Marinenko (1994) has used this method extensively with good results in the former Soviet Union. The surface materials are carefully chosen with reflective properties and the time trace of the initial impulse, time delay gap, and subsequent reflections are analyzed to determine the significance of various surfaces in providing reflected energy, similar to in Figures 8–1a and 8–1b.

Even well-designed environments may have a nonuniform sound field as a result of the geometry and room content. For example, the *Seat-Dip Effect* caused by the absorptive presence of heavily upholstered seating can cause a lessening of energy in the low to mid-frequency region (100 to 400 Hz). The other design elements such as properly angled reflective clouds, or electronic equalization through the use of a properly designed sound reinforcement system, when appropriate, can be useful in compensating for this effect.

A last but extremely important consideration in music hall acoustics is the provision of a sufficiently *Diffuse* sound field. Irregular surfaces such as ornamentation diffuse the sound upon reflection (reflect it in a variety of directions simultaneously) and are used to reduce Acoustic Glare, improve the *Surface Diffusivity Index*, and provide a sense of *Spaciousness* and *Listener Envelopment*. This results in a more effective blending of the sound of ensemble instruments and generally better listening conditions for performers and audience alike.

REVERBERATION TIME

The construction of Boston's Symphony Hall in 1900 marked the first application of Wallace Sabine's research into a measure called *Reverberation Time* (RT).

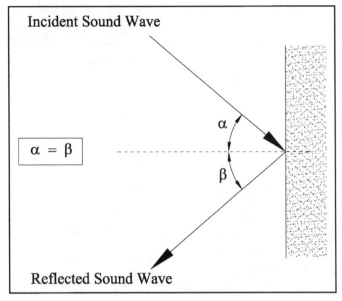

A

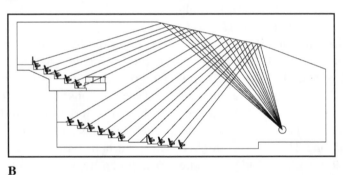

B

Figure 8–2. (**A**) The law of reflection. (**B**) Ray tracing analysis of a stage canopy.

Today, the Boston Symphony Hall, along with the Grosser Musikvereinssaal in Vienna and the Teatro Colon in Buenos Aires, is considered one of the best in existence (Beranek, 2004).

The RT is the length of time in seconds for a sound to decay by 60 decibels. Specifically, it is proportional to the volume of the hall and inversely proportional to the hall's total absorption. Generally, in a well-designed space, the audience provides most of the absorption and the need for additional acoustical treatments, except in the case of variable acoustics, is minimal. Seats should be upholstered, but not too heavily, to replace the absorption of patrons who are not in attendance. A large volume space with minimal sound absorption or occupancy, such as a gymnasium, will have a long RT. In contrast, a library or recording studio with a high level of sound absorption due to an acoustical tile ceiling, carpeting, wall treatments, and shelves full of books will have a short RT. The RT is such an important descriptor that its method of measurement has been standardized for international use (ISO 3382, 1997).

It is interesting to note the relationship between the various styles of music and the performance halls of their day. Beranek (2004) has noted that secular baroque music (1600–1750) tended to be played in palace music rooms and small theaters that were rectangular and full of nonabsorbing ornamentations. RTs were typically less than 1.5 seconds (considered to be a "dry" acoustic). Such halls, with their many nearby sound reflecting surfaces, provided an intimacy and clarity for this highly articulated music. Baroque sacred music covered a more diverse range, but much was played in small chapels or newly constructed Lutheran churches with occupied galleries, resulting in a much more moderate RT (1.6 to 2 seconds) than the cathedral and allowing for the brisk tempo of the fugue. In the Classical period (1750 to 1820), full orchestras with expanding audiences resulted in larger halls with longer RT (1.6 to 1.8 seconds) and more emphasis on fullness of tone. This trend continued through the Romantic period of the late 19th century and the early 20th century with larger halls with even longer RTs (2 second range) and musical compositions that relied less on clarity and more on fullness of tone.

Preferred values of reverberation are given in Table 8-2, taken from several sources including Beranek (2004) and Egan (1988). These values are only approximate because of the large variation in spatial volume associated with facilities, but these tend to reflect the preference of user groups.

The large range of music performed in modern concert halls demands a more variable environment, and modern halls can be designed with variable acoustical

Table 8–2. Desired Reverberation Times (RTs)

Performance	RT (seconds)
Traditional organ music	2.5–5.0
Symphonic repertoire	1.8–2.1
Chamber music	1.6–1.8
Opera	1.3–1.6
Modern music	1.1–1.7
Live theater	0.9–1.4
Lecture or conference	0.6–1.1
Broadcast, recording studios	0.3–0.7

features for different events. These include moveable stage shells, canopies, and reflective ceiling panels to optimize early reflections. This is the application in which well designed and placed variable absorptive elements such as banners, curtains with pleats, and reversible panels can be most useful. Typically, the audience and the upholstered theater seating can provide sufficient absorption to control reverberation within acceptable limits, but these additional treatments can fine tune the reverberation to optimal levels for different musical performances. Truly multipurpose halls incorporate many such features so that a wide variety of entertainment can be provided at a single venue.

KEY POINT

Insufficient reverberation can result in excessive strain on musicians as the orchestra attempts to accommodate.

The value of these features should not be underestimated in terms of workplace comfort, health, and safety. Beranek (2004, p. 5) includes materials indicating that, if a venue has less than a desirable degree of reverberation, it "absorbs and even chokes sound, impedes leisurely tempi and long soaring lines. In response the orchestra's conductors have required endless bow arms of the players and directed them to attack and sustain notes in order to make the music 'sing.'"

MORE COMPLEX REVERBERATION MEASURES

Table 8–3 shows that a superior, a good, and a fair-to-good concert hall can have similar RTs despite the dramatic difference in subjective preference. Clearly, the single measure of RT cannot in itself account for the subjective quality preference of a performance hall. The following is a discussion of some other measures that have been found to useful indicators.

The early decay time (EDT) is based on the initial decay (10 decibels), which is the only part of the decay process that remains audible between rapidly played notes. As such, it tends to correlate better with acoustical quality for symphonic music than RT.

The C80 ratio of early to late sound energy is determined by the energy summed in the first 80 ms as compared to the energy in the remainder of the reverberant sound (Bradley, 1991). This ratio correlates highly with *Clarity* and *Definition*. One reason for the success and lasting usefulness of rectangular music halls is that strong early reflections from side walls and ceiling enhance clarity.

The interaural cross-correlation coefficient (IACC) is a measure of the difference in sound between the two ears with the listener facing the source (Hidaka, Beranek, & Okano, 1995). It correlates well with spaciousness because the sensation of spaciousness depends strongly on early lateral (horizontal) reflections.

The use of sound reinforcement systems to increase loudness is discouraged for most classical or symphonic music concerts, for which the concert hall and its particular acoustical signature are an important part of the performance. Sound reinforcement systems form an integral

Table 8–3. Different quality concert halls but similar Reverberation Times (RT)

Concert Hall	Quality	RT
Symphony Hall, Boston	Superior	1.85
Davies Hall, San Fransisco	Good	1.85
Barbican Large Hall, London	Fair to good	1.7

Note. Data compiled from "Interaural Cross-Correlation, Lateral Fraction, and Low and High Frequency Sound Levels as Measures of Acoustical Quality in Concert Halls," by T. Hidaka, L. L. Beranek, & T. Okano, 1995, *Journal of the Acoustical Society of America, 98*(2), pp. 988–1007. Used by permission.

part of theatrical and modern music productions, which favor venues with relatively dry acoustics. In that case, the sound system becomes part of the performance, adding reverberation or special effects as required, and the hall simply becomes a transparent vehicle to convey the production with as little interference as possible.

MUSIC REHEARSAL SPACES

The primary acoustical goal of a music rehearsal space is to allow the players and teacher to hear each other well without excessive loudness. A second goal is to keep others from hearing them, by providing good sound isolation.

The most common deficiency in the design of music rehearsal spaces is insufficient physical volume or ceiling height. Sound levels can be reduced both by increasing the room volume and by adding acoustically absorptive treatments. The former is the better solution.

Rooms with low ceilings and reflective parallel surfaces make poor rehearsal spaces because the sound and reverberation levels are high. These interfere with the musicians' ability to hear each other well and earplugs may be a necessity. The installation of an absorptive acoustical ceiling and wall panels reduces the sound levels, but larger groups of musicians still can't hear each other well because there are no beneficial early reflections from the ceiling and upper wall surfaces.

An optimal design should consider a physical volume of at least 17 cubic meters per person. Typically, a ceiling height of at least 7 meters is required to achieve sufficient volume so that sound levels are maintained at acceptable levels.

Sufficient volume and ceiling height allow the possibility of providing a well-balanced combination of reflective diffusing treatments to the upper room surfaces to spread sound efficiently around the space and provide a reasonable level of reverberation for good sound quality and sufficient cross-room early reflections to enhance hearing and group playing. There are several suppliers of acoustical treatments specifically for music rooms that have adopted and support this design philosophy.

ANSI S12.60-2002, Acoustical Performance Criteria, Design Requirements, and Guidelines for Schools, suggests for a large core learning area a midband (500 Hz) RT of 0.7 to 1.1 s (ANSI, 2002). This is to ensure good speech intelligibility between the teacher and students. Beranek (2004) indicates that music rehearsal spaces should have RTs on the order of 0.3 to 0.4 seconds less than considered optimal for a performance space, again to enhance intermusician audibility and blend. This implies RTs on the order of 1.2 to 1.7 seconds, typically for acoustic instruments. This issue is made more interesting when modern music teaching is added to the activities. My recent experience indicates that reverberation times in this range can be considered by educators to be too high for activities involving electric bass, keyboards, and drums and RTs closer to the ANSI S12.60-2002 may be more appropriate. A slightly longer RT in the bass frequencies maintains some warmth for the acoustic instruments, but excessive low frequency reverberation can be problematic. A shorter RT in the highest treble frequencies (4000 Hz and 8000 Hz bands) helps reduce the harshness of cymbals without overly affecting the overtones of the brass instruments or violins in these relatively small rooms, effectively providing the excess absorption that the air would provide in the concert venue.

KEY POINT

Music rehearsal and teaching spaces require sufficient physical volume to avoid excessive acoustical volume and the potential for hearing loss. Additional absorptive treatments can be helpful but result in a dry acoustic, and volume levels could still be excessive.

The reverberation spectra for one such relatively small music room (470 m³) are provided in Figure 8–3 before and after

additional absorptive treatments were introduced to control reverberation and reduce the overall sound levels. Because significant additional absorption can be required, it should be distributed as evenly as possible around the walls and ceiling to enhance diffusion and inter-player hearing as much as possible.

ORCHESTRA PITS

Similar factors influence the design of orchestra pits. Bigger (volume) is better, although not as much volume is required as in a rehearsal space because the orchestra pit is coupled to the volume of

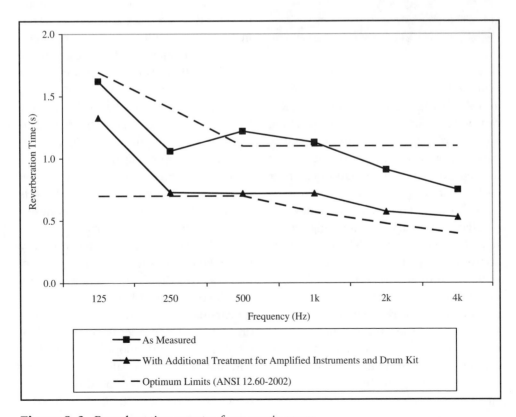

Figure 8–3. Reverberation spectra for a music room.

the main hall, generally through a front of stage opening. A reflective ceiling is preferred for intermusician intelligibility and to propagate sound out of the pit, but there should be sufficient acoustical treatment to allow sound control, and that treatment should be variable, depending on the number and types of musicians.

This can be accomplished through the use of large areas of moveable stage drapery and local treatments around drum kits, for example. The amount of sound propagating into the hall can also be controlled by providing removable panels over some of the exit area. If the pit is too small, flexibility is limited and there may be no way to effectively control either the acoustics or the overall sound levels.

INDIVIDUAL PRACTICE OR TEACHING ROOMS

It would be wonderful if we all had large rehearsal spaces with great acoustics available to use for individual practice or teaching, but of course most teaching spaces are practically and necessarily small. Because teacher and student are located close to each other, they can hear each other well without extensive ceiling reflections, and a high efficiency suspended acoustical tile ceiling (high noise reduction coefficient [NRC] rating) is appropriate. Absorptive wall panels are useful in rooms with no other furnishings, but in many practice rooms most of the wall surfaces are covered with bookshelves and other furnishings, which tend to have the same effect. Interroom privacy is also important, and acoustical doors and sound isolating walls, ceilings, and ductwork should be well considered in the design.

KEY POINT

Variable (changeable) acoustic elements are required for successful multipurpose halls.

WORKPLACE SOUND LEVELS

A thorough analysis and review of the sound levels found on the stages, rehearsal halls, and classrooms of the world is beyond the scope of this chapter, but some of that information has become available to me over the years as an electric guitarist and consulting engineer with access to an integrating sound level meter.

In my experience, it is not uncommon for time averaged sound levels (Leq) in high school music rooms to exceed 85 dBA, depending on class size and room effects, but time averaged sound levels typically do not significantly exceed 90 dBA (Gastmeier, Pernu, & Chasin, 1994). Typical sound levels in an acoustically treated music room are shown in Figure 8–4. Sound levels in a highly reverberant music room or on stage in a rock band can be considerably higher, as can sound levels in small concrete and drywall orchestra pits or basement practice rooms.

In the past, it was difficult to clearly prove damage risk for teachers, for example, because the 90 dBA guideline was not clearly exceeded. For performing or rehearsing musicians, limited exposure times provided another uncertainty. New regulations recently adopted by the Occupational Health and Safety Act (OHSA) in Ontario go further to address these issues as shown in Table 8–4 (OSHA, 1990, Amended 2007).

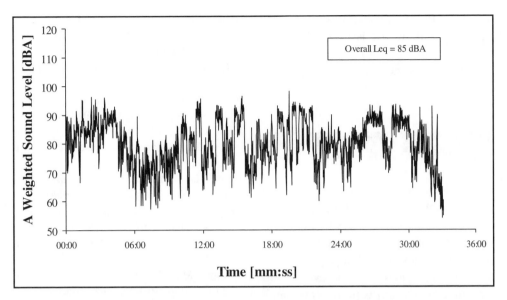

Figure 8–4. Sound levels measured during a high school music class.

Table 8–4. Summary of OHSA sound exposure limits

Previous Regulation		Revised Regulation	
Sound Level (Leq, dBA)	Allowable Exposure (hrs.)	Sound Level (Leq, dBA)	Allowable Exposure (hrs.)
90	8	85	8
95	4	88	4
100	2	91	2
105	1	94	1

Note. From Occupational Health and Safety Act. Revised Statutes of Ontario.

The changes are significant. The combined effect of reducing both the criterion and the exchange rate is to substantially lower the sound level considered acceptable for shorter durations of exposure more typical of a musician's workplace —several hours spent in an orchestra pit, on stage in a club, or in front of a class, for example.

There may still be a reluctance on behalf of regulators, compensation boards, venue operators, and school boards to classify musical workplaces and classrooms as industrial workplaces, but at least these regulations should serve to remind working musicians that their hearing health really is at risk. Musicians should be encouraged to find personal means to address problems and educate themselves about the issue so that they can speak intelligently about it and about appropriate solutions when the opportunity arises.

SUMMARY

Performance and rehearsal spaces are professional workplaces that should be designed with hearing health and safety considerations in mind. A well-designed performance space with adequately sufficient early sound reflections, even sound distribution, and appropriate reverberation greatly benefits the performers as well as the listeners. Acoustic defects such as Standing Waves, Sound Focusing, Flutter Echoes, Acoustic Glare, and Source Shift should be avoided. Variable (changeable) acoustic elements are required for successful multipurpose halls.

Insufficient reverberation can result in excessive strain on musicians as the orchestra attempts to accommodate. Music rehearsal and teaching spaces require sufficient physical volume to avoid excessive acoustical volume and the potential for hearing loss. Additional absorptive treatments can be helpful but result in a dry acoustic, and volume levels could still be excessive.

REFERENCES

American National Standard. (2002). *Acoustical performance criteria, design requirements, and guidelines for schools.* Melville, NY: Acoustical Society of America.

Ando, Y., & Gottlob, D. (1979). Effects of early multiple reflections on subjective preference judgments of music sound fields. *Journal of the Acoustical Society of America, 65,* 524–527.

Beranek, L. L. (1962). *Music, acoustics, and architecture.* New York: Wiley Press.

Beranek, L. L. (1988). *Noise and vibration control.* Washington, DC: Institute of Noise Control Engineering.

Beranek, L. L. (2004). *Concert halls and opera houses.* New York: Springer-Verlag.

Bradley, J. S. (1991). Comparison of a multipurpose hall with three well-known concert halls. *Canadian Acoustics, 19*(2), 3–10.

Campbell, M., & Greated, C. (1987). *The musician's guide to acoustics.* London: J. M. Dent.

Egan, D. M. (1988). *Architectural acoustics.* New York: McGraw-Hill.

Gastmeier, B., Pernu, D., & Chasin, M. (September, 1994). *Occupational noise exposure in the high school music practice room.* Technical paper presented at the 1994 Congress of the Canadian Acoustical Association, Ottawa, Canada.

Hidaka, T., Beranek, L. L., & Okano, T. (1995). Interaural cross-correlation, lateral fraction, and low and high frequency sound levels as measures of acoustical quality in concert halls. *Journal of the Acoustical Society of America, 98*(2), 988–1007

International Standards Organization. ISO 3382, (1997). *Acoustics—Measurement of the reverberation time of rooms with reference to other acoustical parameters.*

Makrinenko, L. (1994). *Acoustics of auditoriums in the public buildings.* Woodbury, NY: Acoustical Society of America.

New York Times, August 10, 2007

Ontario Ministry of Labour Occupational Health and Safety Act (1990). *R.R.O. 1990, Regulation 851; Amended to O. Reg. 629/05.*

9 Inexpensive Environmental Modifications

BY MARSHALL CHASIN

EDITOR'S NOTE

This chapter has been written primarily for musicians and laypersons rather than for hearing health care professionals. The suggestions and modifications that are discussed may be straightforwardly implemented by anyone including musicians, teachers, or concerned parents.

In addition to hearing protection, which is covered in Chapter 6, there are other strategies aimed at minimizing the potentially hazardous effects that loud music can have on hearing. These can be divided into two categories: (a) altering the input, based on loudness perception and improved monitoring; and (b) modifying the listening environment or loudspeaker system.

LOUDNESS PERCEPTION AND IMPROVED MONITORING

The human auditory system, as discussed in Chapter 2, is incredibly complex both in its anatomy and its physiology. A full understanding of its operation involves a number of areas of study including acoustics, psychology, biology, physics, hydrodynamics, electronics, and even mechanisms that are similar to digital computer storage. An interaction between the physical and perceptual qualities of sound gives rise to a number of psycho-acoustic phenomena, including a relationship between the intensity of musical inputs and how loudly they are perceived. The interplay between intensity (a physical measure) and loudness (a perceptual measure) is crucial in determining how an individual selects a "comfortably loud" listening level.

Loudness and Intensity

Intensity, typically measured in decibels (dB), is a purely physical measure that quantifies the level or energy of transmitted sound. There are *sound level meters*, which are devices that can give us precise intensity readings. In contrast, loudness is the subjective perception of intensity and falls along a descriptive continuum between "very soft" and "very loud" and can be further defined in terms of comfort levels. There is no such thing as a "loudness meter." Not surprisingly, there is usually a good correlation between the physical measure of intensity and the subjective sense of loudness, yet there can be some important differences. A primary strategy for hearing loss prevention among those in the performing arts is hinged upon the distinctions between intensity and loudness.

An example of the difference between intensity and loudness is when we are driving in a car while listening to the radio. While driving at a slow speed, we adjust our radio to a comfortable listening loudness and find that it is at an intensity level of 65 dB (if we had a sound level meter and were able to safely measure the sound while keeping our eyes on the traffic). If the speed was increased, because of the greater engine and wind noise, we would need to make corresponding increases to the intensity of the radio to maintain the same level of comfortable listening. Thus, a new sound level reading of intensity may show an increase to 85 dB, although our subjective evaluation of loudness is unchanged and remains "comfortable."

Despite the fact that our auditory system is remarkable and we can discriminate frequency changes of only a couple of Hz, our perception of sound intensity is rather poor. Depending on our listening level and our listening environment, a change of 2 to 3 dB may not even be noticeable. Yet, an increase of only 3 dB in intensity corresponds to a doubling of exposure. For example, if we were to increase the volume on a radio (above 85 dB) by 3 dB, this may generate only a very slight increase in loudness (if any), but will in fact double the potential damage to the auditory system. Conversely, a 3 dB reduction of intensity (e.g., from 100 dB to 97 dB) would have the effect of lowering the risk of damage by half.

There is a direct relationship between sound intensity and sound duration in the determination of the maximum safe dosage for loud sounds. Every 3 dB increase or decrease in exposure (at potentially hazardous intensity levels) will double or halve the damage to hearing. By extention, each 3 dB reduction in intensity allows for a corresponding doubling of exposure duration to produce an equivalent dosage. Following this line of reasoning, a 15 dB reduction (which is found in musician earplugs such as the ER-15, discussed Chapter 6) means that a musician or listener can be exposed 32 times as long before the same damage to hearing occurs.

Improved Monitoring

Selection of a volume setting on any amplifier system, including MP3 players or even hearing aids, depends on many acoustic factors including the intensity, shape, and bandwidth of the frequency response and isolation from background noise. The car example mentioned earlier could be thought of as a case where the environmental wind noise masked or covered over the music from the radio such that it needed to be more intense. Minimizing background noises (such as traffic) may be useful for improved monitoring, which results in a lower listening intensity for a comfortable loudness.

An approach based on monitoring that can help reduce the risk of hazardous noise levels consists of *increasing* the amount of low frequency, bass sounds that a person hears. This may first appear counterintuitive; however, raising the bass setting on an amplifier will lead to an increased sense of loudness that in turn can lead to a reduction in intensity to maintain comfort. For example, at noisy exercise/health clubs or dance studios where instructors are typically exposed for 8 to 10 hours each day, increasing the base (loudness) while decreasing the volume (intensity) can make the listening environment much safer. Thus, with a simple change to the bandwidth of the music, overall intensity can be reduced by 6 to 9 dB, which itself will provide a four- to eightfold increase in the allowable exposure time before damage occurs.

One relatively recent technical innovation is that musicians have started to replace the old style wedge monitors up on stage with custom-made ear monitors (see Chapter 7). These have the advantage of partially isolating the musician from the immediate environment. A picture of an ear monitor is shown in Figure 9–1. The overall intensity is about 6 dB lower when these ear monitors are worn, as compared to the intensity with the wedge monitor speakers. The musician does not need to compete as much with the other sounds in the performing environment. This means that the musicians can be exposed four times as long (6 dB less intense) with these monitors as compared to the on-stage wedge monitors.

SIX ENVIRONMENTAL STRATEGIES

Six inexpensive and expeditious environmental techniques to reduce music exposure along with their rationales are listed below. Their suitability may be dependent on specific characteristics of a particular venue, but they are equally applicable among professionals and amateurs.

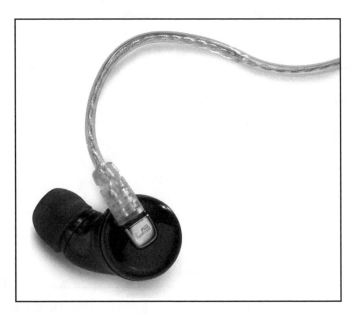

Figure 9–1. Picture of an ear monitor, which replaces the on-stage wedge and sidewash loudspeakers. *Note.* Photograph courtesy of UltimateEars. Used with permission.

Speaker/Amplifier Enclosures Should Be Elevated

Speakers (some with built-in amplifiers) are situated on the stage and can be used both as monitors (where the musician is "downwind") and as amplifiers to improve audibility for the audience. Low frequency (bass) notes can be personified, or thought of, as "lazy" because they always take the "easy route" or path of least resistance. For example, a speaker enclosure that is in contact with the floor will only generate mid- and high frequency energy with any significant force because the low frequency energy will travel into the nearby floor surface (with its lower resistance). As a result, the acoustic low frequency energy would mostly be lost to the audience; this phenomenon is illustrated in Figure 9-2. As a consequence, many sound engineers respond to this loss of the low frequency sound energy by increasing the overall level in order to reestablish the proper sense of loudness. A smart engineer will simply use an equalizer to turn up the volume on those missing lower frequency sounds in order to reestablish a flat response. Unfortunately, for most engineers, this increase in intensity brings with it a greater risk for music induced hearing loss. A simple solution is to elevate the speakers on stands (or even milk crates), which will increase the distance to the floor and thereby increase the resistance for low frequencies. This will subsequently provide the dual benefits of a flatter output response and a lower overall level.

Treble Brass Instruments Should Be on Risers
(or at least not on the playing plane of the other musicians downwind)

Although it may seem to the casual observer that all sounds from a trumpet emanate from its bell, it is only the higher

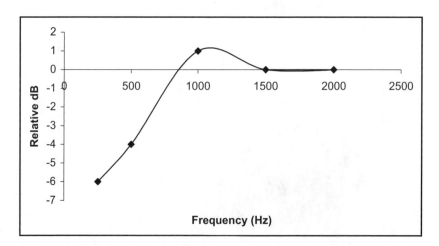

Figure 9–2. Loss of low frequency sound energy due to the loudspeaker enclosure being in contact with the floor. Elevating the loudspeaker will result in a flatter frequency response and an overall lower listening volume, because of improved low frequency monitoring ability.

frequency notes that travel this route. Mid- and low frequency notes tend to "leak" out of the trumpet from all sides. Not only are the higher frequency harmonic notes the most intense within the trumpet's spectrum, but they also travel in an almost "straight line" manner like a laser beam and emanate along the plane of the instrument. This is also true of the human vocal tract. Raising the playing position of trumpeters allows the higher frequency notes to pass over the heads of the other musicians located downwind. The highly directional pattern emanating from a trumpet bell for higher frequency sounds, as compared with the relatively nondirectional pattern for lower frequency sounds, is shown in Figure 9–3. Placing the trumpets on risers (whether it is a high school band class, a jazz band, or a classical symphony) can reduce music exposure from this source by up to 8 dB. This strategy relates closely to that of elevating loudspeaker enclosures, which

was discussed previously. Loudspeakers are also directional for higher frequency sounds; therefore, placing them closer to ear levels will provide musicians with a better sound (i.e., a flatter response) at an overall lower intensity level because the volume does not need to be adjusted as high.

The Orchestra/Band Should Be Set Back from the Edge of the Stage

Placing the band away from the edge of the stage allows both the incident sound of instruments (or voices) and the higher frequency sounds that are reflected off the stage floor to better reach the audience. Sound engineers typically have considerable challenges with room acoustics given that there is far greater lower frequency energy compared to high frequency energy present at the back of

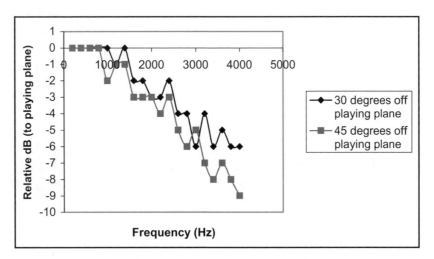

Figure 9–3. The difference in decibels between a measurement on the playing plane of the trumpet, 30°, and 45° off axis (normalized to the playing plane). Lower frequencies are nondirectional (i.e., not affected by playing plane), whereas the converse is true for higher frequency sounds. The higher frequencies tend to emanate from the trumpet bell much like a laser beam.

concert halls. Setting the band back from the edge of the stage will provide an increase in high frequency energy (up to 6 dB) to help resolve this problem. This high frequency emphasis, caused by the presence of unoccupied floor space on stage, functions as an "acoustic mirror" and emphasizes the higher frequency sounds, as shown in Figure 9–4. The overall intensity level of the playing/amplification will be lower and the music will sound better. This translates into reduced risk of hearing damage to the audience and less arm and wrist strain for the musicians on stage.

Treble Stringed Instruments Should Be Away from Overhangs

This environmental modification is based on the fact that higher frequency sounds, by virtue of their short wavelengths, are easily absorbed by acoustically treated surfaces (see also Chapter 8). High frequencies don't like small spaces and tend to be easily absorbed with a resulting attenuation, or loss of energy. This can have important ergonomic consequences for violinists and violists. These musicians, if placed under an overhang (such as a music pit), have to more greatly exert themselves to compensate for the lost high frequency energy that has been absorbed. Figure 9–5 shows the deleterious effect of placing violinists under a poorly constructed orchestral pit overhang. Not only will the overall intensity level of this large musical section be greater, but there is a significant risk of arm or wrist damage for these musicians. Moving violinists and violists away from an overhang will reduce both the overall intensity of their instruments and the risk of injury from physical strain.

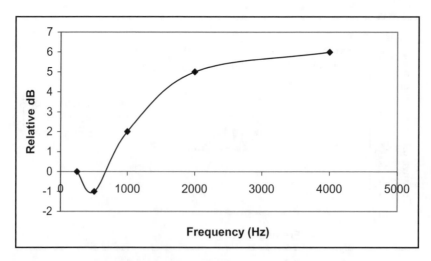

Figure 9–4. A high frequency sound enhancement can be achieved by setting the orchestra or band 2 meters back from the lip of the stage. Because of shorter wavelengths, the mid- and high frequency sound energy adds constructively with its reflection off the lip of the stage.

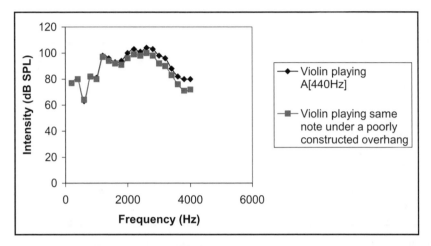

Figure 9–5. A poorly constructed orchestral pit overhang absorbs the higher frequency components such that a violinist needs to play harder in order to reestablish the higher frequency harmonic energy. Wrist and arm problems can ensue.

The Use of Baffles

Camp and Horstman (1992) demonstrated that the effect of baffles is limited beyond a distance of approximately 7 inches. The manner in which incident sounds bounce off walls, ceilings, floors, and other obstructions compromises the attenuating effect of baffles. Also, because longer wavelength low frequency sounds are not as easily obstructed as are shorter wavelength high frequency sounds, baffles more effectively attenuate higher frequencies; in fact, it is possible to achieve up to 17 dB of high frequency attenuation with virtually no attenuation below 1000 Hz. Given the limited benefits of baffles, in terms of providing insufficient attenuation and imposing impractical proximity constraints on musicians, they have not found widespread use. Figure 9–6 is from Camp and Horstman (1992) and shows a typical attenuation of a Lucite baffle. However, attenuations on the order of 8 to 10 dB are commonplace, and although baffles do not achieve results as impressive as other methods of reducing sound levels, they ought not to be dismissed. In conjunction with other techniques (such as hearing protection), baffles can be a significant and inexpensive device in the toolbox. Recall that even a 3 dB attenuation can cut the potential damage in half, a 6 dB attenuation can cut the damage to one quarter, and a 9 dB attenuation can cut the damage to one eighth. The attenuation characteristics of baffles are also related to their mass, physical thickness, and method of construction; for example ¾ inch Lucite baffles will attenuate less than 2 inch wooden ones. The angle of baffles can also alter the amount of energy that reflects back to the musician. A vertical orientation will maximize the reflected energy to the musicians' ear, whereas one that is oriented 30° away (or towards) the musician would have less deleterious reflection (while still maintaining the attenuation for those musicians downwind).

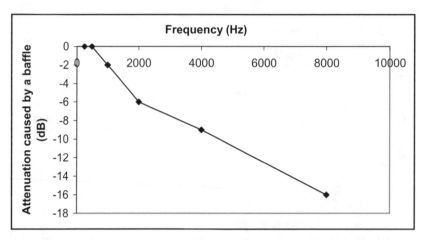

Figure 9–6. Attenuation characteristics of a Lucite baffle showing poor low frequency attenuation. *Note.* Based on data from "Musician Sound Exposure during Performance of Wagner's Ring Cycle," by J. E. Camp & S. W. Horstman, 1992, *Medical Problems of Performing Artists*, 7(2), pp. 37–39. Used with permission.

Changing the Location of Certain Instruments

In many cases, there are no reasons— outside of historical protocol—why the positioning of certain instruments cannot be changed. This is true of many musical genres, including classical, rock, and pop. For example, in many modern shows, it is not uncommon for the percussion section to be in a separate room linked via video monitors and headphones. Trumpets, typically one of the most intense instruments in any musical ensemble, are further amplified in many shows. Relocating the trumpets in front of other instruments would not usually alter the music heard by the audience, yet significant reductions in music-related hearing loss could be realized by musicians who would otherwise be downwind. Thus, there are distinct advantages of not having trumpet sections in their traditional orchestral positions at the rear.

Changing the orientation of certain cymbals in the percussion section may also be beneficial. Depending on the cymbal configuration, the sound may emanate from them in a directional manner. This implies that a slight movement in cymbal orientation and/or location may significantly reduce the overall sound level and the overall annoyance of neighboring musicians.

SUMMARY

There are a number of strategies to reduce the potentially damaging effects of loud music on hearing. The strategies and environmental modifications discussed in this chapter are inexpensive and can be implemented in a wide range of performing and teaching venues. Environmental alterations or modifications to the room, to the location of the orchestra or band,

and in the loudspeaker system can all provide additional relief while maintaining optimal music quality and acceptance by both performers and their audiences.

Acknowledgments. Some parts of this chapter were presented at the Music—Safe and Sound Conference: European Forum on Hearing Conservation for Professionals in Music and Entertainment, Dortmund, Germany, 2007.

REFERENCE

Camp. J. E., & Horstman, S. W. (1992). Musician sound exposure during performance of Wagner's Ring Cycle. *Medical Problems of Performing Artists*, 7(2), 37–39.

10 Hearing Aids and Music

BY MARSHALL CHASIN

INTRODUCTION

As an auditory stimulus, music presents some challenging problems to both hearing aid design engineers and hearing health care professionals. The following discussion equally concerns the issues involved in fitting hearing aids to musicians as well as nonmusicians who are music enthusiasts. In many cases, as will be seen, success will not hinge upon deriving an ideal set of elctroacoustic parameters, but rather on whether hearing aid manufacturers are willing and capable of providing subtle changes based on the unique characteristics of an individual. In order to understand the changes necessary for music as an input to a hearing aid or a cochlear implant, four primary physical differences between speech and music need to be understood. They are (a) the long-term spectrum of music versus speech, (b) differing overall intensities, (c) crest factors, and (d) phonetic versus phonemic perceptual requirements of different musicians.

Music Long-Term Spectrum versus Speech Long-Term Spectrum

Speech is derived from the complex interaction of respiratory, phonatory, and articulatory structures and is comprised of a long-term spectrum that is well defined and typically language independent. In addition to the contributions of the vocal tract, music is derived from many sources with specific resonance characteristics: percussive instruments (e.g., drums); woodwind or brass instruments acting as quarter wavelength resonators (e.g., clarinets) or one half wavelength resonators (saxophones); and stringed instruments (such as violins and guitars) that act as half wavelength resonators. All of these sources can be amplified or unamplified. Depending on the music and instruments involved, even unamplified sources can produce high intensity sounds. Moreover, some instruments can produce both high and low frequency spectrum emphasis. Unlike speech, music is highly variable and the concept of a "long-term music spectrum" is poorly defined. There is simply no music "target" as there is for amplified speech. Chapter 12 covers many of these concepts in more depth.

Differing Overall Intensities

At one meter, average speech measures 65 dB SPL (RMS) and has peaks and valleys of about 12 to 15 dB in magnitude. Although human variability provides for a wide variety of vocal qualities and characteristics, the considerable physical similarities across human lungs and vocal tracts results in a rather narrow long-term spectrum of approximately 30 to 35 decibels. In contrast, depending on the music, instruments can generate very soft sounds (20–30 dB SPL from brushes on a jazz drum) to dangerously loud sounds (over 120 dB SPL from brass instruments in Wagner's Ring Cycle). At 100 dB, the dynamic range of music as an input to a hearing aid is far greater than that of speech.

Crest Factors

The crest factor is the difference in decibels between the peak (most intense part) of a waveform and its average or root mean square (RMS). The RMS value corresponds with one's perception of loudness—the subjective attribute correlating with intensity. For speech, the RMS is about 65 dB with a crest factor of approximately 12 dB. This is well known in the hearing aid industry and this characteristic of speech is utilized in hearing aid compression circuitry and test systems. Among the more significant factors giving rise to the 12 dB crest factor in

speech is the damping or loss of energy that is inherent to soft walled vocal tracts. Before a spoken word is heard, the vocal energy passes by a soft tongue, soft cheeks and lips, and a nasal cavity full of soft tissue and occasionally some other foreign "snotty" materials. These soft tissues dampen the sound such that the peaks are generally only 12 dB more intense than the average intensity of the speech. In contrast, a trumpet has no soft walls or lips. Thus, most musical instruments are less damped and produce "peakier" sound compared to speech. Crest factors of 18 to 20 dB are not uncommon for many musical instruments. Compression systems and detectors that are based on peak sound pressure levels may have different operating characteristics for music versus speech. In other words, music may cause some compression systems to enter its nonlinear phase at a lower intensity than what would be appropriate for that listening condition.

Another aspect of the crest factor for instrumental music is that it has ramifications for specifying both OSPL90 and gain. Loudness discomfort levels for speech are typically used for setting the OSPL90 for a hearing aid, yet music and speech have differing crest factors. The peaks of instrumental music are 6 dB higher than for speech (given the same RMS value) because the crest factor for instrumental music is 6 dB greater than that for speech (12 dB vs. 18 dB). In order to prevent a tolerance problem for instrumental music, the OSLP90 for a "music program" therefore needs to have a 6 dB less intense OSPL90 than that for speech. And, given similar compression characteristics between music and speech, this implies that the gain for a music program should be 6 dB lower than the gain for a broadband speech channel as well.

Phonetic versus Phonemic Perceptual Requirements

There are important distinctions between that which is heard by way of physical vibrations in the air (phonetic) and the perceptual needs or requirements of the individual or group of individuals (phonemic). These terms derive from the study of linguistics, but have direct applicability here. Despite the fact that the long-term speech spectrum for all languages has most of its energy in lower frequency regions and less in the higher frequency regions (i.e., phonetic manifestation), the clarity (e.g., as measured by word recognition scores or speech intelligibility indices) is generally derived from mid- and high frequency regions. This mismatch between energy (phonetic) and clarity (phonemic) is complex but well understood in the field of hearing aid amplification.

Although there are common frequency ranges that listeners depend upon to perceive speech, the requirements for musicians can be quite different. Some musicians have a greater reliance on lower frequency sounds. For example, clarinetists are typically satisfied with their tone only if the lower frequency inter-resonant breathiness is at a certain level, despite the fact that the clarinet can generate significant amounts of high frequency energy. This is in sharp contrast to violinists, who need to hear the magnitude of higher frequency harmonics before they can judge that a good sound has been achieved. The clarinet and the violin both have similar energy spectra (i.e., similar "phonetics"), but dramatically differing uses of the sound (i.e., "phonemics").

These four differences between the physical properties of speech and music can now serve as the basis for differing electroacoustic settings of a hearing aid for speech and music as inputs.

KEY POINT

The energy distribution of music differs from noise by spectral shape, overall intensity, and the crest factor.

"THE FRONT END"—PEAK INPUT LIMITING LEVEL IN HEARING AIDS: NOT A "PROGRAMMING ISSUE"

This is the most important of all factors in selecting a set of electroacoustic parameters that are optimal or near optimal for listening to amplified music through a hearing aid. Many hearing aids on the market have a front-end limiter or clipper that prevents sounds above 85 to 90 dB SPL from effectively *entering* the hearing aid. This should not be confused with output limiting. There is a trend within the industry, however, toward manufacturing hearing aids that have peak input limiting levels that are on the order of only 95 to 100 dB SPL. Historically, this has been quite reasonable because the most intense components of shouted speech are approximately 85 to 90 dB SPL. In addition, manufacturers of digital hearing aids want to ensure that the analog-to-digital (A/D) converter is not overdriven. The argument is that any sound above about 90 dB SPL is not speech (or speechlike), and as such, the limiter will function as a rudimentary noise reduction system. However, music is generally much more intense than 85 to 90 dB SPL and would therefore be limited or distorted at the front end of the hearing aid. Modern hearing aid microphones can certainly handle up to 115 dB SPL without appreciable distortion so there is no inherent reason (other than historical and limiting an input to a poorly configured A/D converter) for having such an input limiting level set so low. Once intense inputs are limited and distorted at the front end of the hearing aid, regardless of the music program that is applied later on, music will never be clear or of high fidelity. A patient may request "programming" changes because of poor hearing aid performance with music. However, the solution is rarely confined to programming and has more to do with the intense inputs prior to the A/D converter.

There are techniques to avoid this front-end distortion problem and, depending on the implementation, may use a compressor to "sneak" under the peak limiter with expansion after the limiter point in the hearing aid. Hearing aids are also available with very high peak input limiting levels. The challenge is analogous to an airplane that must travel under a low bridge: unless the bridge is raised or the plane travels near the ground, problems will occur.

Research has shown that anything below a peak input limiting level of 105 dB SPL will cause a deleterious distortion for music regardless of what program(s) come later in the hearing aid (Chasin, 2003, 2006b; Chasin & Russo, 2004). A "quick and dirty" clinical test of a hearing aid to determine if its front end clips or distorts loud music is to set the output high (>115 dB) and the gain low (5-8 dB). In a hearing aid test box, apply an intense signal (e.g., 100 dB SPL); there should not be any peak clipping (because the output is set >115 dB SPL). If there is a high level of distortion (i.e., >10%), then the culprit is most likely a front end or peak input limiting level that is too low to handle (intense) music. Results for five commercially available hearing aids are shown in Table 10-1 (Chasin, 2006a).

An example of a hearing aid that had a very high peak input limiter was the K-AMP. Another example is the Venture digital platform with the HRX (Headroom Extension) feature enabled from Sound Design Technologies (formerly a division of Gennum Corporation). (An earlier version served as the basis for the Digi-K hearing aid). The peak input limiting level is not a requirement of ANSI S3.22-1996 (R. 2003) or any of the proposed updates and may therefore not appear on hearing aid specification sheets. However, this information is typically available upon request from hearing aid manufacturers.

Table 10–1. Harmonic distortion (in percent) at 1600 Hz for five commercially available hearing aids with two input levels of 90 dB SPL and 100 dB SPL. Aid #2 performed the best.

	Aid #1	Aid #2	Aid #3	Aid #4	Aid #5
90 dB input	10	3	16	21	16
100 dB input	22	5	54	58	57

Note. From "Can Your Hearing Aid Handle Loud Music? A Quick Test Will Tell You," by M. Chasin, 2006, Hearing Journal, 59(12), pp. 22–24. Used with permission of The Hearing Journal and its publisher, Lippincott Williams & Wilkins.

SOME STRATEGIES IF THE PEAK INPUT LIMITING LEVEL IS TOO LOW

Turn Down or Dampen the Input

If a patient has a hearing aid with a peak input limiting level that is too low for music, one strategy would be to turn down the input (e.g., home stereo or MP3 system) and turn up the gain of the hearing aid. This would allow "the plane to fly under the bridge," as discussed earlier. Another approach simply uses a *resistive network* just after the hearing aid microphone that "fools" the hearing aid into thinking that the input is 10 to 12 dB less intense. Typically, this network is only engaged (with a button) for the music program. Figure 10-1 shows the effect of a resistive network. It should be noted that the output is 10 to 12 dB softer only because the input is 10 to 12 dB softer, with no change in gain. Most manufacturers can accomplish this resistive network so that the interested clinician can use this approach with

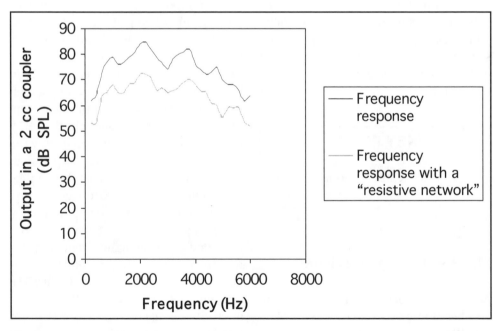

Figure 10–1. Output in a 2 cc coupler showing both the unaltered frequency response and one with a specially built resistive network designed to bias the microphone by making it 10 to 12 dB *less* sensitive. This would allow 10 to 12 dB greater headroom for more intense inputs such as music, *without affecting gain. Note.* From "Can Hearing Aids Handle Loud Music?" by M. Chasin, 2007, *Canadian Hearing Report, 2*(2), pp. 29-33. Used with permission of Canadian Hearing Report.

their favorite hearing aids. The question is not "Which is the best hearing aid for music?" but rather "Who is the most flexible hearing aid manufacturer that can implement circuit changes such as a resistive network?"

Other techniques that are not as elegant, but still effective, include placing a Band-aid–like cover over the hearing aid microphone(s) to fool the hearing aid into thinking that the input is lower (because of the attenuation from the Band-aid). The gain may or may not need to be increased to compensate because music is generally more intense than speech. The effect of using commercially available adhesive tape (e.g., Scotch tape) over the hearing aid microphone(s) can also be very useful. A very uniform attenuation of 5 dB from 200 Hz to 4000 Hz can be accomplished with a slight increase in attenuation above 4000 Hz. This simple clinical "Scotch tape trick," which does not require changing gain settings, can provide an additional 5 dB of headroom input before distortion is encountered.

KEY POINT

A less sensitive microphone (or front end) may be better for loud music.

Fletcher-Munson Revisited

Another approach derives from the Fletcher-Munson curves (Fletcher & Munson, 1933), also known as *equal loudness curves*. These equal loudness contours indicate that even those with a moderate sensorineural hearing loss will retain a normal loudness function for inputs that are sufficiently intense—that is, for higher stimulus levels, a given sensorineural hearing loss may be less of a problem. This is why people with a mild high frequency sensorineural hearing loss, common with music induced hearing loss, may not require any "correction" to their hearing and rarely would require any equalization (specific boosting of certain frequency ranges) to optimally hear the music. This is also the rationale for why modern level-dependent hearing aids provide significant gain for quiet sounds, and substantially less gain for louder sounds. Many musicians with significant sensorineural hearing loss, especially those who are exposed to sound levels in the 80 to 100 dB range while performing, typically require only a modest degree (e.g., 15–20 dB) of high frequency amplification. These musicians are ideal candidates for wearing nonoccluding BTE hearing aids when playing louder music. However, if the nonoccluding BTE hearing aids have a broadband microphone, then the front end of the hearing aid can be overdriven. A solution is to use a high frequency emphasis microphone in conjunction with the nonoccluding BTE hearing aids. In this scenario, the low frequency sounds would be lost through the nonoccluding ear canal, but unlike the condition with a broadband hearing aid, the more intense lower frequency components would not overdrive the front end or cause higher frequency distortion. The frequency response would be the same for these nonoccluding BTE hearing aids regardless of the type of microphone used, but the distortion would be dramatically lower (i.e., the microphone would be damped for most intense low frequency sounds below 700–800 Hz) for the aid with the high frequency microphone.

KEY POINT

When playing or listening to loud music, a person with a moderate sensorineural hearing loss may only require 10 to 15 dB of gain.

Turn the Directional Microphone Around

Finally, for those who wear BTE hearing aids that use a directional microphone, another trick may be helpful. Directional microphones are found in almost all BTE hearing aids as well as in many smaller custom styles. These microphones are designed to suppress noise if it is coming from the rear direction. Directional microphones, in combination with a binaural fitting and the use of an assistive listening device (such as an FM system), would optimize many hearing aid fittings, especially under noisy conditions. The trick involves turning the BTE hearing aid around—the earmold will still fit nicely into the ear, but the tubing in the earhook has been twisted 180° around so that the front of the hearing aid faces to the rear. This is especially practical for hearing aid wearers with long hair for whom the cosmetic consequences would remain invisible. This works because the ports of the directional microphone in the hearing aid will be reversed so that sound from the front will be suppressed. As a result, the hearing aid microphone that receives the louder music is tricked to be less sensitive, which leads to the net effect of raising the limiter bridge.

It should be noted that this only works if the hearing aid uses directional microphones and not two omnidirec-

tional microphones. In the case of two omnidirectional microphones, the processing occurs after the digitization of the signal, so it would not be useful for minimizing distortion caused by intense musical inputs (B. Rule, personal communication, 2008).

ONE CHANNEL MAY BE BEST FOR MUSIC

In sharp contrast to what is typically appropriate for amplifying speech (especially in noise), one channel (or if linear processing, many channels with the same compression ratios and kneepoints) appears to be optimal for hearing music. The relative balance between the lower frequency fundamental energy and the higher frequency harmonics is crucial for listening to most types of music. High fidelity music is related to many parameters, one of which is the audibility of the higher frequency harmonics at the correct amplitude. Poor fidelity can result from the intensity of these harmonics being too low or too high. A multichannel hearing aid that uses differing activation points and differing degrees of compression for various channels runs the distinct risk of severely altering this important low frequency (fundamental)/high frequency (harmonic) balance. Subsequently, a music program within a hearing aid should be comprised of one channel, or equivalently, a multichannel system where all compression parameters are set in a similar fashion. It has been suggested that in some bass-heavy conditions, a two-channel system may be useful with the lower frequency channel set at 500 Hz and greater attenuation at higher input levels (L. Revit, personal communication, 2004).

COMPRESSION

The clinical rules of thumb for setting compression parameters for speech are rather straightforward and any introductory textbook on audiology covers this. The compression detectors are set based on the crest factor of speech, which, as stated earlier, is approximately 12 dB (i.e., the peaks are 12 dB more intense than the RMS). For speech, compression systems function to limit overly intense outputs and to ensure that soft sounds are heard as quiet (but not too quiet) sounds and intense sounds are heard as intense (but not too intense) sounds. In short, these systems take the dynamic range of speech (30–35 dB) and alter it to correspond with the dynamic range of the hearing impaired individual. Furthermore, there is no inherent reason why a wide dynamic range compression (WDRC) system that works well for a patient with speech as input should not also work well for musical inputs. However, the dynamic range of music is typically much greater than that of speech (i.e., 80–100 dB vs. 30–35 dB). Nevertheless, clinically it is observed that no major changes need to be made because the more intense components of music are just in a different part of the input-output operating characteristic of the compression function. The difference lies in whether the compression system uses a peak detector or an RMS detector. If the compressor uses an RMS (or average intensity) detector, then no changes need to be made for a music program. However, if the hearing aid utilizes a peak detector to activate the compression circuit, for a music program the detector should be set about 5 to 8 dB higher than for speech. This is related to the larger crest factor of music (18 dB vs. 12 dB for speech), and care should be taken that these peaks should not activate the compression circuit prematurely.

FEEDBACK REDUCTION SYSTEMS

In most cases, given that the spectral intensity of music is greater than for speech, feedback is not an issue. The gain of the hearing aid for these higher level inputs is typically less than for speech. However, if feedback reduction is required, or the feedback circuit cannot be disabled in a music program, then those systems that utilize a gain reduction method would be the best. The two other feedback management approaches, namely notch filtering and phase cancellation, may create a dilemma. It is not so much that gain reduction is the proper approach as it is that the other two approaches can cause major problems for listening to and playing music. In the notch filtering approach, the center frequency of the filter may "hop" around, searching for the feedback, thereby causing a blurry sound. This has been called the *frequency-hopping artifact* (Chung, 2004). The phase cancellation approach uses a technique where a signal is generated that is 180° out of phase with the feedback. Although this works well for speech and the majority of hearing aid manufacturers use such a technique, the narrow bandwidth harmonics of music (because there is minimal damping) can, and do, confuse the hearing aid into suppressing the music. In addition, if the harmonic is of short duration, the created cancellation signal can become audible and is heard as a brief "chirp." Two approaches have been used to remediate this. One is to limit the feedback detector to the very high frequency range where the musical harmonic structure is inherently less intense, or to use a two-stage phase cancellation technique using both fast and slow attack times. However, if at all possible, disabling any feedback reduction system would be the optimal approach for listening or playing music.

KEY POINT

If possible, disable the feedback and noise reduction program.

NOISE REDUCTION SYSTEMS

As is the case for feedback reduction systems, it would be best to disable the noise reduction system when listening to music. Typically, the signal-to-noise ratio is quite favorable, so noise reduction would not be necessary. However, for some hearing aids, the noise reduction system cannot be disabled, and because the primary benefit for noise reduction systems is to improve listening comfort rather than reduce noise, choosing an approach for music that has minimal effect may be beneficial for a music program. It should be noted that, unlike compression systems that use a fast attack time and slow release time, noise reduction systems use opposite time constants —a slow attack time and a fast release time. With slow attack times, noise reduc-

tion systems will not be as deleterious to the perception of music as they would be for the perception of speech because music has a higher modulation rate and will typically not allow the noise reduction algorithm to engage as frequently.

SUMMARY: THE MUSIC PROGRAM

A music program, or a set of optimal electroacoustic parameters for enjoying music, would include:

1. A sufficiently high peak input limiting level so more intense components of music are not distorted at the front end of the hearing aid.
2. If playing in an intense environment, even for those with significant sensorineural hearing loss, a nonoccluding BTE *and* a high frequency emphasis microphone.
3. Either a single channel or a multichannel system in which all channels are set for similar compression ratios and kneepoints.
4. A compression system (similar to the speech-based compression system) with an RMS detector compression scheme that has a kneepoint 5 to 8 dB higher if the hearing aid uses a peak compression detector.
5. OSPL90 and gain, for the instrumental music that is 6 dB less intense than for broadband speech.
6. A disabled feedback reduction system, or a feedback reduction system that uses gain reduction or a more sophisticated form of phase feedback cancellation (either one with short and long attack times or one that only

operates on a restricted range of frequencies such as over 2000 Hz).

7. A disabled noise reduction circuit, although because of a long attack time and a short release time, this circuitry may rarely be activated for many forms of music.

REFERENCES

American National Standards Institute (1996). Specification of hearing aid characteristics (ANSI S3.22-1996). New York: Acoustical Society of America.

Chasin, M. (1996). *Musicians and the prevention of hearing loss.* San Diego, CA: Singular.

Chasin, M. (2003). Music and hearing aids. *Hearing Journal, 56*(7), 36-39.

Chasin, M. (2006). Can your hearing aid handle loud music? A quick test will tell you. *Hearing Journal, 59*(12), 22-24.

Chasin, M. (2006). Hearing aids for musicians. *Hearing Review,* 13(3), 24-31.

Chasin, M. (2007). Can hearing aids handle loud music? *Canadian Hearing Report, 2*(2), 29-33.

Chasin, M., & Russo, F. A. (2004). Hearing aids and music. *Trends in Amplification, 8*(4), 35-47.

Chung, K. (2004). Challenges and recent developments in hearing aids: Part 1. Speech understanding in noise, microphone technologies and noise reduction algorithms. *Trends in Amplification, 8*(3), 83-124.

Fletcher, H., & Munson, W. A. (1933). Loudness, its definition, measurement and calculation. *Journal of the Acoustical Society of America, 5*(1), 82-108.

Kent, R. D., & Read, C. (2002). *Acoustic analysis of speech* (2nd ed.). Clifton Park, NY: Delmar Thomson Learning.

11 Cochlear Implants and Music

BY HUGH J. McDERMOTT

Over 25 years ago, when commercial development of electronic devices intended to restore hearing to deaf people commenced, it would have seemed unlikely that such devices would ever be the topic of a chapter in a book concerned mainly with music. However, recent technological advances are showing some promise for improving the representation of musical sounds in patterns of electrical nerve stimulation. Early devices were designed to stimulate the auditory nerve in people with total or profound deafness in both ears. The most successful of those devices delivered electric stimuli to neurons from a number of discrete locations in the cochlea, which is the inner ear structure that normally converts the mechanical vibrations of sound into perceptible neural activity. Although only the array of electrodes in such devices is placed inside the cochlea, the term *cochlear implant* is now commonly used to describe any hearing prosthesis system of this type.

Initially, cochlear implants were designed primarily as aids to speech-reading ("lip-reading"). By stimulating the auditory nerve electrically, they pro-duced hearing sensations that provided their users with limited awareness of environmental sounds as well as information about speech that is difficult to perceive visually, such as voicing. Although several early cochlear implants attained these goals, large improvements in performance followed the subsequent development of better ways to process sound signals for delivery to the auditory nerve (McDermott, 2006). Now that there are well over 100,000 users of cochlear implants worldwide, expectations of the quality of auditory perception available from electric stimulation are relatively high. Most recipients of modern devices can readily understand speech without visual cues, at least in favorable listening conditions. Therefore, there has been considerable growth in interest recently about the perception of music and other sounds with electric stimulation. In this chapter, experimental results related to music perception will be discussed, and some potential opportunities for improved performance in future will be presented. First, though, the topic will be introduced with an outline of how existing cochlear implant systems function.

117

KEY POINT

Cochlear implants provide people having severe or profound hearing impairment in both ears with some ability to perceive sounds by means of direct electrical stimulation of the auditory nerve.

HOW COCHLEAR IMPLANTS WORK

As explained in previous chapters, normal hearing is the perception of rapid pressure fluctuations in air. Such pressure changes are converted into mechanical vibrations by the tympanic membrane (*eardrum*) that is located in the ear canal, where it separates the outer ear from the middle ear. These vibrations are coupled to a membrane-covered opening in the cochlea by a chain of small bones in the middle ear. The cochlea is filled with fluid, in which waves are created by the vibratory motion imparted to its membranous lining. Inside the cochlea are approximately 15,000 hair cells that detect the wave motion and convert it into neural activity. This activity is processed and relayed by a series of neural networks leading to patterns of excitation in the auditory cortex. In the brain this neural activity elicits the sensation of hearing sounds.

Permanent hearing loss can be the result of many diverse causes. Sensorineural impairment usually involves damage to hair cells and neurons, and can be a consequence of exposure to excessively loud sounds. Diseases such as meningitis, medical treatment with certain antibiotic drugs, and head trauma can also cause sensorineural hearing loss. For mild or moderate degrees of impairment, acoustic hearing aids are the most common and effective remedy. However, amplification of sounds is often not adequate to restore hearing in many cases of more severe loss. In such cases the damage to hair cells may be so extensive that stimulating them acoustically or mechanically cannot elicit hearing sensations that are sufficiently loud, completely intelligible, and easily discriminated. Cochlear implants partly solve this problem by stimulating neurons electrically, thus bypassing the dysfunctional transduction of acoustic vibrations.

A block diagram of a modern cochlear implant system appears in Figure 11–1. The components shown above the horizontal dashed line are in the sound processor, which is worn externally in existing implant systems. Sounds enter a microphone, usually located near the pinna (external ear) and are converted into electrical signals. These signals may be processed in various ways to reduce noise, compensate for level variations, or emphasize some frequencies over others. The short-term spectra of the input signals are then estimated using either a Fourier transform or a bank of band-pass filters. The frequency components of the signals are separated by this process so that they can be assigned to appropriate electrodes in the cochlea. The acoustic levels of the signal components are converted into levels suitable for electric stimulation of the auditory nerve. Digital data specifying these parameters of the stimuli are encoded and transmitted across the intact skin via an inductive radio-frequency link.

The implanted parts of the system are shown below the horizontal dashed line.

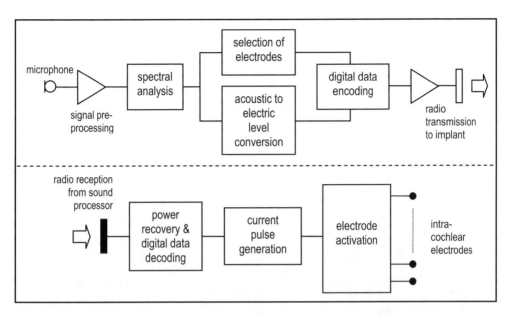

Figure 11–1. Block diagram showing the main functional elements of a modern cochlear implant system. Components shown above the horizontal dashed line are in the externally worn sound processor, whereas components below the line are in the implanted device. Sounds enter the system via the microphone (*top left*) and are processed to extract and encode important information. Digital data specifying the required pattern of stimulation are transmitted across the skin to the implanted device, which generates electric current pulses to stimulate the auditory nerve via an array of electrodes in the cochlea (*bottom right*).

The data from the sound processor are received from the transcutaneous inductive link and decoded to obtain the electrode selection and level parameters. At the same time, electric power is recovered from the transmitted signal to generate the stimuli so that the implant is not required to contain a battery. In most existing systems, the stimuli comprise brief current pulses that are delivered to the electrodes in rapid succession. The pulses stimulate surviving auditory neurons along much of the length of the cochlea.

The relationship between the sounds picked up by the microphone and the stimuli delivered to the cochlea is complex and varies considerably among systems that are presently available. The overall function of one widely used system, known as ACE (Vandali, Whitford, Plant, & Clark, 2000), is illustrated in Figure 11-2. The upper panel of that figure shows the spectrogram of a flute playing an arpeggio. The sequence of notes was G4, B4, D5, G5. These notes have fundamental frequencies of approximately 392, 494, 587, and 784 Hz, respectively. The spectrogram shows the frequency content (in kHz, vertical axis) as a function of time (horizontal axis). Dark areas represent components having relatively high acoustic energy. For instance, the first note had components at 392 Hz and

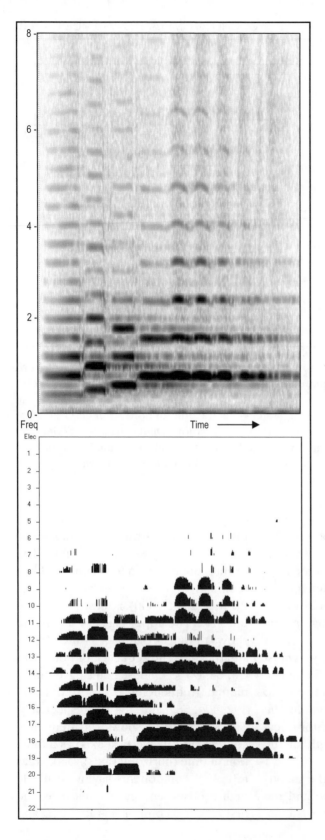

Figure 11–2. Spectrogram (*upper panel*) of the sounds made by a flute playing an arpeggio, and the corresponding stimulation from a cochlear implant (*lower panel*). The spectrogram shows frequency (*in kHz, vertical axis*) versus time (*horizontal axis*), and the dark areas indicate frequency components having relatively high intensity. The output of the implant is plotted on the same time scale, whereas the vertical axis shows electrode number. The most apical electrode is at the bottom of the axis and is activated by the lowest frequency components in the incoming sound (around 250 Hz), whereas the most basal electrode at the top of the axis is activated by frequencies around 7.4 kHz. The allocation of acoustic frequencies to electrodes is not linear, so the vertical axes in the two panels are not identical. The notes played sequentially by the flute were G4 (fundamental frequency: 392 Hz), B4 (494 Hz), D5 (587 Hz), and G5 (784 Hz). *Note.* Figure modified from C. M. Sucher, personal communication, August 1, 2007.

its harmonics, which are at multiples of the fundamental frequency (i.e., 784, 1176, 1568, 1960 Hz, etc.). The darkness of the band at 784 Hz indicates that it was the most intense component of that note. The lower panel of Figure 11–2 shows the output of a 22-electrode cochlear implant in response to the flute sound. The electrodes (vertical axis) are assigned to the acoustic frequencies such that electrode 1, which is at the basal end of the cochlea, is activated mainly by frequencies around 7.4 kHz (top of axis), whereas electrode 22, which is at the apical end of the cochlea, is activated by frequencies around 250 Hz (bottom). This allocation of frequencies to electrode positions corresponds approximately to the filtering function of the normal cochlea, and is known as tonotopic organization. However, the frequencies are not usually assigned to the electrodes linearly. Therefore, the vertical axes of the upper and lower panels in the figure are not identical. In the lower panel, the height of the bars at each electrode position indicates the intensity of the electrical stimulation. The time axis is the same as in the upper panel. Thus, for the first note, most stimulation occurred on electrode 18, which is activated by frequencies around 750 Hz. Many other electrodes were also activated by this acoustic signal, but the harmonic structure of the sound is much less distinct than in the spectrogram. In general, the representation of the flute sounds by the pattern of electric stimuli appears somewhat coarse. As will be discussed later, the crude conversion of acoustic signal components into neural activation patterns by existing cochlear implant systems can result in poor perception of music by many of their users.

MUSIC APPRAISAL BY COCHLEAR IMPLANT RECIPIENTS

In recent years, several publications have reported on the subjective appraisal of musical sounds by implant users (McDermott, 2004). As with many other investigations into the performance of cochlear implants, the findings of these studies can be difficult to summarize accurately because of factors such as differences in the experimental methods and materials used and the large variability among the responses of subjects. However, a fair generalization of most of these reports is that adult implant users do not find music as pleasant to listen to as adults with normal hearing. For example, one study obtained a rating of overall pleasantness on a scale of 0 to 100 from subjects listening to recordings of eight different musical instruments (Gfeller, Witt, Woodworth, Mehr, & Knutson, 2002). The recordings were representative of brass, woodwind, and stringed instruments, including the piano. On average, the implant users gave ratings that were about 17 points lower than the subjects with normal hearing.

Another study compared the ratings of quality assigned to musical sounds by subjects with cochlear implants and subjects who used conventional acoustic hearing aids (Looi, McDermott, McKay, & Hickson, 2007). In addition, a group of hearing aid users who subsequently received cochlear implants provided quality ratings both before and after implantation. Interestingly, their ratings were significantly higher with use of the implant compared with preoperative use of hearing aids. This was consistent with the results from the other two subject groups, which showed a trend for higher quality ratings from the implant users than the hearing aid users.

Several experiments have found that ratings of quality or pleasantness by implant users tend to be higher for musical sounds that are relatively simple. For example, one study that included a comparison among classical, country-western, and pop musical styles found that classical music was less liked than the other two styles (Gfeller, Christ, Knutson, Witt, & Mehr, 2003). In another study, music played on single instruments received higher quality scores, on average, than music involving multiple instruments played simultaneously (Looi et al., 2007).

KEY POINT

Technological advances have enabled most implant recipients to understand speech satisfactorily and to recognize many other types of sound, at least in favorable listening conditions.

When cochlear implant recipients have been asked to compare their experience of listening to music through the device with their recollection of listening to music preoperatively with acoustic hearing, a common finding is that the performance of implant systems is disappointing to many of their users. For instance, one study reported that only about 21% of implant users enjoyed music and sought opportunities to listen to it (Leal et al., 2003). However, of the subjects in the same group who could recall listening to music before their hearing deteriorated to levels that justified implantation, 41% stated that they enjoyed music at that time. In contrast, a more recent study found that 70% of implant users reported listening to music regularly (Brockmeier et al., 2007). This is consistent with the statement in another publication that approximately one third of implant users tended to avoid listening to music because of its aversive sound quality when heard through the device (Gfeller et al., 2000).

WHY IS THE QUALITY OF MUSICAL SOUNDS POOR?

Many studies have investigated the ability of implant users to perceive certain fundamental characteristics of musical sounds, such as rhythm, pitch, and timbre (McDermott, 2004). In general, these studies have shown that information about rhythm is relatively well preserved in the patterns of electrical stimulation produced by implant systems. This is not surprising, because users of modern implant devices can usually understand speech adequately, and it is known that this ability depends heavily on the perception of coarse temporal cues. Such cues are similar to those that convey rhythmic aspects of music. For instance, in one typical study of rhythmic pattern discrimination, 24 of 29 implant users obtained scores of at least 90% correct (Leal et al., 2003).

Experiments investigating the ability of implant listeners to perceive pitch are inherently more complicated. In particular, there are important distinctions between being able to determine that two pitches are different, being able to state which pitch is higher, and being able to estimate the size of the musical interval between the pitches. Nevertheless, all published studies concur on the poor ability of implant users to discriminate pitch relative to the typical ability of listeners with normal hearing. In one recent study, subjects were asked to rank the pitch of pairs of sung vowels that had been recorded with fundamental frequencies separated by either one semitone or six semitones. Normally hearing subjects obtained average scores of 81% and 89% correct for the two intervals, respectively, whereas the corresponding scores for implant users were only 49% and 60% correct (Sucher & McDermott, 2007). The latter scores seem particularly low in consideration of the fact that a score of 50% would be expected with merely random responses in this type of experiment.

The ability to identify common melodies is a basic skill of music perception. Although a few well-known tunes may be recognizable by their distinctive rhythm, the ability to perceive accurately at least the changes in pitch within melodies assists greatly with their identification. Given the experimental results mentioned above, it is not surprising that implant users' recognition of familiar melodies is often poor, especially if rhythmic or verbal cues are not present. In one representative report, the average score for a group of 49 implant recipients was only 19% correct for a set of 12 common tunes, whereas a group of normally hearing listeners scored 83% correct on the same test (Gfeller, Turner, et al., 2002).

KEY POINT

Performance of existing cochlear implant systems is generally not satisfactory for listening to music, although most implant recipients can perceive musical rhythm adequately.

The perception of timbre (i.e., the quality that enables sounds to be distinguished even when they have identical pitch and loudness) is more difficult to measure experimentally. Several studies have addressed this topic by means of tests that involve recognition of sounds, or, more specifically, identification of musical instruments using acoustic signals only. In one experiment, 51 users of cochlear implants and 20 listeners with normal hearing were asked to identify eight different instruments (Gfeller, Witt, et al., 2002). The subjects' responses were limited to a set of 16 possible choices. The implant users obtained an average score of only 46.6% correct, whereas the corresponding score for the normally hearing listeners was 90.9%. Not only was the implant users' mean score significantly lower than that of the subjects with normal hearing, but their responses were also less consistent. In particular, they frequently confused instruments across different musical "families," such as woodwind and strings, whereas the few errors made by the normally hearing subjects were usually within an instrumental family.

IMPROVING MUSIC PERCEPTION WITH COCHLEAR IMPLANTS

It may seem that the results summarized briefly above are somewhat pessimistic concerning the ability of implant recipients to accurately perceive and appreciate music, or to sing or play a musical instrument proficiently. However, at present there are three major avenues of research that may lead to improvements in the performance of implant devices specifically for listening to musical sounds.

First, much of the published experimental data has been obtained from studies with adults, many of whom were profoundly hearing impaired for some years before receiving an implant. Over at least the past 20 years, there has been substantial growth in the number of children receiving implants, and a decrease in the earliest age at which implantation is considered appropriate. It is plausible that young children may obtain more information about music through implant systems than adults because of the inherently greater plasticity of the developing brain. Furthermore, it is likely that children may enjoy listening to music through an implant more than adults who acquired hearing impairment later in life because they would not be influenced by any previous experience of musical qualities perceived with acoustic hearing (Mitani et al., 2007). Future research will reveal whether profoundly deaf children implanted at an early age can obtain more information and enjoyment from musical sounds than adults who lost their acoustic hearing a relatively short time before receiving an implant.

A second area of research that may enhance performance of implant systems for listening to music involves the development of improved sound processing techniques. As outlined above, one of the main problems with existing devices is that pitch information is not delivered to the residual auditory neurons by electric stimulation in a way that enables pitch to be perceived reliably and accurately. Many researchers have assumed that this may be largely a consequence of employing a constant rate of pulsatile stimulation. In existing systems, pitch information is encoded partly in the temporal pattern of amplitude modulations carried on the pulse trains conveyed to each intraco-chlear electrode, and partly in the spatial pattern of stimulation across the array of electrodes (see Figure 11–2). Both these types of pitch information have intrinsic shortcomings that reduce the ability of implant recipients to perceive adequate detail in the pitch of musical sounds. For example, pitch is conveyed by the frequency of amplitude modulations up to a limit of only about 300 Hz, and there is little convincing evidence that changes in the place of stimulation convey pitch changes that are orderly in the musical sense (McDermott & McKay, 1997). Nevertheless, it is possible that a different combination of spatial and temporal patterns of stimulation, or enhancements of those patterns, would convey more pitch information. Unfortunately, results published so far have shown only modest improvements in performance with use of such schemes, although some modifications of the general principles underlying the way stimulation is generated seem promising (Laneau, Wouters, & Moonen, 2006; Vandali et al., 2005).

The third area of current research that is particularly relevant to music perception concerns bimodal stimulation. As perceptual results with cochlear implants have improved over time, the criteria for implantation candidacy have been relaxed progressively. It is now not unusual for implant recipients to have usable acoustic hearing in one or both ears. In certain cases, hearing can be preserved to some extent in the ear that is implanted, especially if a relatively short electrode array is used (Gfeller et al., 2007). More commonly, however, most acoustic hearing sensitivity is available in the ear opposite to the one receiving the implant. Recent research has investigated the perception of sounds, including music, when signals are presented to the listener via both modes of auditory stimulation. Because the configuration of the hearing loss in these listeners almost always indicates better sensitivity at low frequencies than at high frequencies, the acoustic signal provides mainly low pitched sensations, whereas the implant provides information about a wide range of acoustic frequencies, including relatively high frequency components that may not be audible acoustically even after amplification.

Some results of a recent study that aimed to determine whether bimodal stimulation was beneficial for music perception are summarized in Figure 11–3.

Ten subjects who used both cochlear implants and acoustic hearing aids participated in three experiments. In the first experiment, they were asked to identify each melody from a set of seven familiar melodies (e.g., "Happy Birthday"), presented without words and without rhythmic cues. Each of the melodies was presented eight times in a random order. In the second experiment, the subjects were required to identify each of 16 types of sound from a closed-set list. The sound types were representative of speech, single musical instruments, musical ensembles, and environmental noises. Each

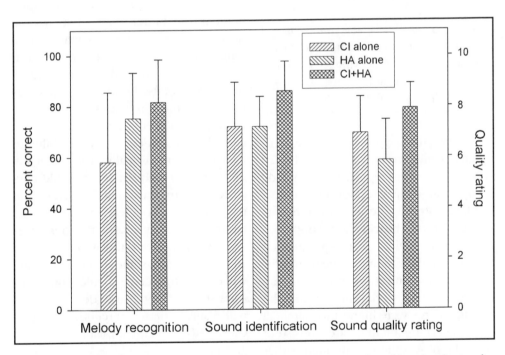

Figure 11–3. Results of three experiments with 10 recipients of cochlear implants who were also users of acoustic hearing aids. In each experiment, the listeners were tested in three conditions: when using the cochlear implant (CI) alone; when using the hearing aid (HA) alone; and when using both devices simultaneously (CI+HA). Results averaged across the subjects are shown for each experiment and each listening condition, with error bars indicating one standard deviation. The melody recognition and sound identification tests were scored as percentages of correct responses (*left axis*), whereas the sound quality ratings were obtained on a scale of 1 to 10, with higher numbers indicating better quality (*right axis*).

sound type was presented four times from a total of 64 different recordings in a random order. The same acoustic signals were used in the third experiment, which sought sound quality ratings from the subjects. A rating scale was presented to each subject in the form of a visual analog, from which a number in the range of 1 to 10 was obtained for each sound. The three experiments were conducted separately with each subject for each of three listening conditions: cochlear implant alone, acoustic hearing aid alone, and both devices together.

KEY POINT

Large benefits are available immediately to those implant recipients who have sufficient acoustic hearing to be capable of perceiving sounds using acoustic and electric signals simultaneously.

As shown in Figure 11–3, the experimental results averaged across the 10 subjects revealed a regular trend. Melody recognition was poorest for the cochlear implant listening condition, and was higher for the hearing aid condition. However, the highest score was obtained for the bimodal condition. The results for the sound identification and quality rating experiments were similar in that the average scores were highest for bimodal listening. These findings are consistent with the observation mentioned earlier about pitch information; such information is not conveyed accurately by existing implant systems, but is usually present in the low frequency signals available to implant recipients who have usable acoustic hearing. In addition, sound quality is generally improved when residual acoustic hearing is combined with electric stimulation.

SUMMARY

Although cochlear implants have demonstrated great success in enabling people with severe or profound bilateral hearing impairment to understand speech, the performance of existing devices for listening to music is less satisfactory. In particular, the ability of most implant recipients to perceive musical pitch and timbre is limited. It is probable that continuing improvements in device design and signal processing will lead to better perceptual performance. It is also possible that children implanted at an early age will learn to appreciate and comprehend music better than adults whose hearing has been severely impaired for a long time before implantation. However, at present the most promising area of research is focused on the simultaneous use of cochlear implants and acoustic hearing aids. Recent studies have provided considerable evidence that the ability to hear sounds acoustically, even over a limited range of frequencies, can add constructively to the auditory perception provided by a cochlear implant. As the technology evolves and the outcomes improve, it is likely that more children and adults with some acoustic hearing will choose to receive cochlear implants. Almost certainly these developments will result in better perception of musical sounds for many implant users.

REFERENCES

Brockmeier, S. J., Grasmeder, M., Passow, S., Mawmann, D., Vischer, M., Jappel, A., et al. (2007). Comparison of musical activities of cochlear implant users with different speech-coding strategies. *Ear and Hearing, 28*(Suppl. 2), 49S–51S.

Gfeller, K., Christ, A., Knutson, J., Witt, S., & Mehr, M. (2003). The effects of familiarity and complexity on appraisal of complex songs by cochlear implant recipients and normal hearing adults. *Journal of Music Therapy, 40*(2), 78–112.

Gfeller, K., Christ, A., Knutson, J. F., Witt, S., Murray, K. T., & Tyler, R. S. (2000). Musical backgrounds, listening habits, and aesthetic enjoyment of adult cochlear implant recipients. *Journal of the American Academy of Audiology, 11*(7), 390–406.

Gfeller, K., Turner, C., Mehr, M., Woodworth, G., Fearn, R., Knutson, J., et al. (2002). Recognition of familiar melodies by adult cochlear implant recipients and normal-hearing adults. *Cochlear Implants International, 3*(1), 29–53.

Gfeller, K., Turner, C., Oleson, J., Zhang, X., Gantz, B., Froman, R., et al. (2007). Accuracy of cochlear implant recipients on pitch perception, melody recognition, and speech reception in noise. *Ear and Hearing, 28*(3), 412–423.

Gfeller, K., Witt, S., Woodworth, G., Mehr, M. A., & Knutson, J. (2002). Effects of frequency, instrumental family, and cochlear implant type on timbre recognition and appraisal. *Annals of Otology, Rhinology and Laryngology, 111*(4), 349–356.

Laneau, J., Wouters, J., & Moonen, M. (2006). Improved music perception with explicit pitch coding in cochlear implants. *Audiology and Neuro-Otology, 11*, 38–52.

Leal, M. C., Shin, Y. J., Laborde, M.-L., Calmels, M.-N., Verges, S., Lugardon, S., et al. (2003). Music perception in adult cochlear implant recipients. *Acta Otolaryngologica, 123*(7), 826–835.

Looi, V., McDermott, H., McKay, C., & Hickson, L. (2007). Comparisons of quality ratings for music by cochlear implant and hearing aid users. *Ear and Hearing, 28*(Suppl. 2), 59S–61S.

McDermott, H. J. (2004). Music perception with cochlear implants: A review. *Trends in Amplification, 8*(2), 49–82.

McDermott, H. J. (2006). Cochlear implants. In M. Akay (Ed.), *Encyclopedia of biomedical engineering* (pp. 186–204). Hoboken, NJ: Wiley.

McDermott, H. J., & McKay, C. M. (1997). Musical pitch perception with electrical stimulation of the cochlea. *Journal of the Acoustical Society of America, 101*(3), 1622–1631.

Mitani, C., Nakata, T., Trehub, S. E., Kanda, Y., Kumagami, H., Takasaki, K., et al. (2007). Music recognition, music listening, and word recognition by deaf children with cochlear implants. *Ear and Hearing, 28*(Suppl. 2), 29S–33S.

Sucher, C., & McDermott, H. (2007). Pitch ranking of complex tones by normally hearing subjects and cochlear implant users. *Hearing Research, 230*, 80–87.

Vandali, A. E., Sucher, C., Tsang, D. J., McKay, C. M., Chew, J. W., & McDermott, H. J. (2005). Pitch ranking ability of cochlear implant recipients: A comparison of sound-processing strategies. *Journal of the Acoustical Society of America, 117*(5), 3126–3138.

Vandali, A. E., Whitford, L. A., Plant, K. L., & Clark, G. M. (2000). Speech perception as a function of electrical stimulation rate: Using the Nucleus 24 cochlear implant system. *Ear and Hearing, 21*(6), 608–624.

12 Music for the Audiologist

BY MARSHALL CHASIN AND DORAN HAYES

Without explicitly recognizing it, audiologists have all of the tools for the understanding and analysis of music. In some cases any limitation can be traced to lack of application of a concept and in other cases it is merely terminology. The musical notes versus the frequency in Hz is one such area.

LETTERS AND FREQUENCIES

Musicians use the letters A, Bb, C, whereas audiologists would say 440 Hz, 466 Hz, and 524 Hz. According to the situation and information required in both cases, this may tend to be an oversimplification. Depending on the musical instrument, the note A may have a fundamental (or tonic) on A, but also a range of higher frequency harmonics and overtones whose location and intensities define the musical instrument. Similarly, stating that a certain note (or vowel) is sung at 440 Hz ignores the fact that there is a rich harmonic structure that occurs at the higher frequencies. Accepting this limitation, a notation that has received widespread acceptance is to state the note as A[440 Hz] or more simply as A[440]. This means that

the A on the second space of the treble cleff has a frequency of its fundamental of 440 Hz. Some notes along with their frequencies are given in Figure 12-1.

A convenience of the musical letter terminology is that octaves have the same letter notation—an octave higher than A is A. And a convenience of the frequency notation is that a doubling of the frequency number is one octave higher—880 Hz is one octave above 440 Hz. Clearly, the frequency notation can be more accurate, but within any one cultural style of playing, the letter terminology can be more than sufficient and more innately understood.

KEY POINT

A convenient notation uses both the musical note and its fundamental frequency.

LETTERS AND INTENSITIES

Another notational difference between music and the field of audiology is the specification of loudness and the actual

129

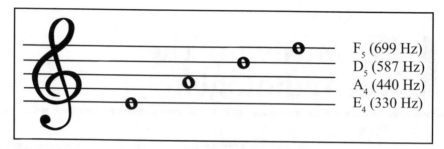

F$_5$ (699 Hz)
D$_5$ (587 Hz)
A$_4$ (440 Hz)
E$_4$ (330 Hz)

Figure 12–1. Several notes shown on a treble cleff along with their frequencies. *Note.* From *Musicians and the Prevention of Hearing Loss* (1st ed.), by M. Chasin, 1996, Clifton Park, NY: Delmar Learning. Reprinted with permission of Delmar Learning, a division of Thomson Learning.

intensity range. Musicians speak in terms of a note being *pianissimo* or *forte*, whereas an audiologist might refer to the level of intensity of a note as being 45 dB SPL or 105 dB SPL. Both are correct despite the slightly more accurate use of the decibel measure for the intensity of the sound. Of course, the reference to a note being pianissimo or *pp* refers to the loudness and not the intensity, but given this difference and the limitations of comparison of a perceptual and a physical measurement, the usage can still be fairly accurate. Musicians around the world can easily play a passage denoted as *mezzo forte* or *mf* with similar intensities because of an underlying familiarity of what the perceived intensity should be. Table 12-1 shows the approximate relationship over a number of musical instruments and styles for a stated loudness level and its corresponding intensity range.

Table 12–1. The approximate relationship between a musician's loudness judgment and the physical intensity measured in decibels (SPL)

Loudness Level	Intensity (dB SPL)
ppp	30–50
pp	45–55
p	50–60
mf	55–75
f	70–80
ff	80–90
fff	90–110

Note. From *Musicians and the Prevention of Hearing Loss* (1st ed.), by M. Chasin, 1996, Clifton Park, NY: Delmar Learning. Reprinted with permission of Delmar Learning, a division of Thomson Learning.

A BIT OF ACOUSTICS

Like all tubes and chambers, musical instruments behave acoustically as resonators. Resonators are structures (e.g., tubes) that serve to amplify sounds that are near the characteristic or resonant frequency. In some cases, the resonant frequency of the tube can be changed either by physically elongating it (such as a trombone) or by covering holes (like a clarinet). And similar to the human vocal tract, these resonators can be classified

Table 12–2. Examples of musical instruments that behave primarily as either a quarter wavelength or a half wavelength resonator

Quarter Wavelength Resonators	Half Wavelength Resonators
clarinet	saxophone
trumpet	oboe
trombone	guitar
tuba	violin
French horn	flute

as quarter wavelength, half wavelength, and Helmholtz resonators. Table 12–2 lists some musical instruments that are considered quarter wavelength and half wavelength resonators.

Quarter Wavelength Resonators

A quarter wavelength resonance occurs whenever a tube has one "open" end and one "closed" end. These occur often and are typically first studied at the high school level. If one pinches a straw at the bottom and blows across the top of the straw, one can hear a unique frequency that is governed only by the length of the straw. And if someone had strong enough lungs, blowing harder would elicit an additional frequency at exactly three times the frequency of the previous one. This is one important feature of a quarter wavelength resonator–successive resonances are at odd-numbered multiples of the resonant frequency, so that no matter what the tonic note is in this type of resonator, other harmonics can be heard.

We see this in behind-the-ear hearing aid acoustics: the hearing aid receiver tubing + earhook + earmold tubing length combine to generate a resonance at about 1000 Hz. Because the hearing aid is closed at the receiver end and open at the end of the earmold, this functions as a quarter wavelength resonator. There are successive "tubing-related" resonances at 3000 Hz and 5000 Hz—or at the odd-numbered multiples of 1000 Hz. In a behind-the-ear hearing aid electroacoustic response there are also resonances in between these wavelength resonances and these are related to the mechanical properties of the hearing aid receiver. Prior to the mid-1980s hearing aids typically used either class A or class B output stages having a mechanical receiver-related resonance at 2000 Hz, but since the advent of the class D output stage, most receivers possess a 2700 to 3000 Hz resonance and may be coincidental with the second mode of the tubing-related resonance at 3000 Hz.

The formula for a quarter wavelength resonator is given by:

$$F = (2k - 1)v/4L$$

Where,
  F = frequency (Hz)
  v = speed of sound
  L = length of the tube
  k = mode or resonance number

The term $(2k - 1)$ is merely a convenience to show that the resonant frequency F not only occurs at $v/4L$ but also at $3v/4L$ and $5v/4L$. Specifically, if $k = 1$, then the term $(2k - 1)$ is simply 1. If $k = 2$ (the second mode of resonance) then the term $(2k - 1)$ is 3 and so on. This formula is also used in speech acoustics and explains why for the vowel [a] as in *father* where the mouth is closed at the vocal

chords and open at the open lips, the resonant pattern of [a] has odd-numbered multiples of the primary resonance 500 Hz.
The 500 Hz can be calculated from the
above formula and is based on the length
of the human vocal tract (about 17 cm).
Subsequent vocal tract resonances (also
called *formants*) are at 1500 Hz (3 × 500
Hz), at 2500 Hz (5 × 500 Hz), and so on.

Clarinets and trumpets are closed at
the lips and open at the other end and as
such behave primarily as quarter wavelength resonators. Other than the fundamental (e.g., A[440]), there are inherent
resonances from these instruments at
1320 Hz (i.e., 3 × 440 Hz) and 2200 Hz
(5 × 440 Hz). Figure 12–2 shows that the
"length" of the clarinet is from the mouthpiece down to the first noncovered hole.
The length below the noncovered hole
does not contribute to the acoustics of
the instrument.

KEY POINT

Clarinets and brass instruments have
odd-numbered multiples of its fundamental frequency.

One aspect of having odd-numbered
multiples of the fundamental or primary
resonance is that in each octave there is
less energy than if there were resonances
at integer numbers of the fundamental
(e.g., violin). The harmonic structure is
less dense for a quarter wavelength resonator than for a half wavelength resonator. Another aspect of quarter wavelength
resonators is that they have a "register key"
and not an "octave key." In the clarinet
the register key increases the frequency
of the note by three times the fundamental, which is in line with the expectation

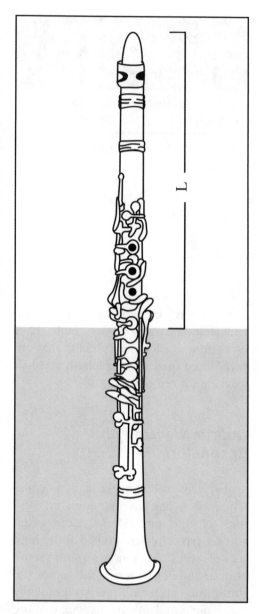

Figure 12–2. The "length" of the clarinet
is from the mouthpiece down to the first
noncovered hole. The region below the
first noncovered hole (shaded in light
gray) does not contribute to the pitch.
Note. From *Musicians and the Prevention
of Hearing Loss* (1st ed.), by M. Chasin,
1996, Clifton Park, NY: Delmar Learning.
Reprinted with permission of Delmar
Learning, a division of Thomson Learning.

of all quarter wavelength resonators. When one plays middle C (concert) on a clarinet the note is 262 Hz, and when the register key is depressed, the note changes to high G [784], which is almost exactly 3×262 Hz. Essentially G[784] is one and one half octaves above concert C [262].

Half Wavelength Resonators

Unlike the quarter wavelength resonators that require a closed end and an open end, half wavelength resonators occur in tubes that are either closed at both ends or open at both ends. Flutes and piccollo function as half wavelength resonators that are open at both ends and violins and guitars function as half wavelength resonators that are closed at both ends. In the stringed instrument category, it is the string that is held rigidly at both ends.

The formula for a half wavelength resonator is given by:

$$F = kv/2L$$

Where again,
  F = frequency (Hz)
  v = speed of sound
  L = length of the tube
  k = mode or resonance number

In this formula, the higher frequency harmonics are merely integer multiples of the primary or fundamental frequency or the tonic. In a one half wavelength resonator instrument such as the flute or violin, the first resonance above concert C[262] would be one octave higher at C[524]. The next would be an octave higher again at C[786], and so on but always remaining the tonic. One half wavelength resonator instruments can have

"octave keys" where their use increases the frequency by exactly one octave (a doubling of frequency). Figure 12–3 shows the clarinet (a quarter wavelength instrument) and a flute (a half wavelength instrument) playing the same *concert* note (G[392]), normalized for playing intensity, demonstrating the differing resonant structures.

Conical Instruments Are Really Half Wavelength Resonators

For reasons beyond the scope of this book, it turns out that conical or gradually flaring tube instruments also behave as half wavelength instruments. The oboe and saxophones are closed at the mouthpiece end and open at the other end, but because of their natural conical flare of the tube, they behave acoustically as if they are half wavelength resonator instruments. Both the oboe and the saxophone have an octave key that serves to double the frequency of playing.

KEY POINT

Stringed instruments as well as the saxophone and oboe have integer multiples of their fundamental frequency.

An aspect of all half wavelength resonator instruments is that the harmonic structure is denser than that of an equivalently sized quarter wavelength instrument. Within each octave, there are two points of energy (at the octaves), whereas for quarter wavelength instruments there is only one (or stated differently, two points of resonant energy every octave and one half).

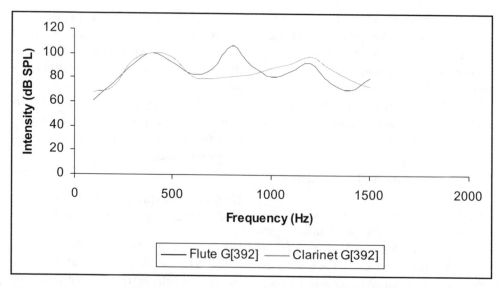

Figure 12–3. This shows the clarinet (a quarter wavelength instrument) and a flute (a half wavelength instrument) playing the same *concert* note (G[392]), normalized for playing intensity, demonstrating the differing resonant structures. The flute has twice as many resonances in any given frequency range as does the quarter wavelength resonator, the clarinet.

Volume-Related and Mechanical Resonances

Other than the two wavelength-related resonances (quarter and half) whose behavior can be ascertained from the end (or boundary) conditions of the tube and the length of the tube, there are resonances that are derived from the volume of air or mechanical characteristics of the wood of the instrument. These non-wavelength resonances are primarily found below 2000 Hz but can be seen as small magnitude ones in the higher frequencies. We have all placed a tuning fork on our knee and then turned around and placed it on the blackboard. While in contact with the blackboard, the tuning fork is much louder—we are driving the natural resonance of the blackboard, which is in the frequency region of the

tuning fork sound. This natural resonance has to do with the size of the board and the material that it is made of.

> ### KEY POINT
>
> Instruments have a "fat" part that is difficult to play quietly.

Musical instruments understandably have these volume- or material-related resonances that serve to enhance the intensity of certain frequencies that are within the amplifying range of the resonance. A flute has a mechanical natural resonance at 880 Hz (which is coincidentally an A), and it is very difficult to play this note quietly. Musicians would refer to this as the fat part of their instrument and with training and skill can learn to harness this natural resonance and shape their musical selections with well-controlled intensity dynamics.

Percussive Instruments

Percussive instruments generate sounds by having a sudden hit of a structure or string. The result can be very tonal or atonal depending on the nature, composition, and shape of the instrument being hit. A characteristic of all percussive instruments is that the resulting sound is broadband in nature and has significant energy in the higher frequencies. It is best to consider the case of a waveform in the time domain. When a percussive instrument is hit, there is a "sudden" change in pressure to a much higher one in a short period of time. If you think about this in terms of the resulting wavelength, this first quarter of the wavelength (from quiet to an intense level), being very sudden, is also very short temporally. Therefore, the entire wavelength would be short as well indicating a high frequency sound. You cannot have a low frequency sudden sound. That is why all sounds in languages of the world that have plosives (e.g., aspiration, affricates, clicks, and pops) are high frequency.

KEY POINT

Percussion has significant high frequency sound energy.

This of course does not mean that all of the sound of that percussive instrument is high frequency. A bass drum has a significant amount of high frequency energy because it is hit suddenly, but also has a significant amount of low frequency energy because of the large surface area of the drum head and large volume of trapped air, which possesses a low frequency resonance.

SUMMARY

Musicians use the notes ranging from A to G along with sharps and flats, and audiologists use frequencies measured in Hz. A convenient notation is a combination of the two—A[440]—meaning that the fundamental (or tonic) of the note A is at 440 Hz. The nature of the higher frequency harmonic structure resulting from the played fundamental note will depend on the acoustic characteristics of the instrument. Instruments that are tubelike and are closed at the mouthpiece and open at the other end are considered to be quarter wavelength resonators and as such will have additional higher frequency resonances at odd-numbered multiples of the fundamental. The first additional higher frequency resonance of these instruments would be at three times (an octave and one half) the frequency of the fundamental. Examples of these instruments are the clarinet and the brass instruments. Instruments that are either closed at both ends (e.g., stringed instruments) or open at both ends (such as the flute) are considered half wavelength resonators and will have higher frequency resonances at integer multiples of the fundamental. The first additional resonance with these instruments will be one octave higher than the fundamental. Half wavelength resonator instruments can have an octave key, whereas quarter wavelength resonator instruments can have a register key (one and one half octaves). Some instruments that are closed at one end and open at the other still behave like half wavelength resonators, and these are those instruments that have a conical flare such as the oboe and the saxophone. The nature of the material, the shape, and the size of the instrument may also yield frequency regions that enhance the intensity of the sound. In the flute, this region is at 880 Hz, and is called the fat region.

13 Human Performance Approach to Prevention: Occupational Darwinism

INTRODUCTION

The last decade of neurobiological research has elucidated the mechanisms of musical perception, sensorimotor integration, and movement control, and the deleterious effects of traumatic stress (van der Kolk & McFarlane, 2006). The application of this knowledge in the treatment of musicians and the prevention of hearing loss is profound.

The effect on hearing of overexposure to noise is well understood, and strategies to reduce sound exposure at the source along with personal hearing protection are standard clinical practice. Musicians have a large stake in their physical and psychological health in order to perform at their optimal level throughout their careers.

This chapter will attempt to integrate these new concepts in order to prevent human performance-related occupational health problems as early as possible.

ALLOSTASIS AND ART

Unlike most occupational health problems, the issue of prevention of hearing loss among musicians serves as an example in which the individual's dependence upon hearing throughout a career is the paramount principle of prevention. This concept linking excessive sound exposure and the performance of musical art challenges the clinicians to not only provide services after the damage is done, but intervene in such a way as to optimize human performance.

The original idea of homeostasis implies that there is an optimal and safe sound exposure to music. However, a new framework of thinking called *allostasis* or *constancy through change* brings into question how the mind and body of a musician anticipate and adapt to the demands of the performance of music (Sapolsky, 2004). Furthermore, when the demands exceed the physiologic capabilities, a stress response is created resulting in what is termed an allostatic overload.

KEY POINT

Excessive sound exposure and musical performance are linked, and when demands exceed physiological capabilities, there can be allostatic overload.

The natural history of sound exposure in a musician's career begins usually at an early age, often paralleling that of the development of speech and language skills. Enhancement of musical performance skills often accelerates to peak performance in early childhood and adolescence. This is in sharp contrast to the average industrial worker, who takes on a job in his 20s and changes very little after that time.

BEETHOVEN AND BODY MAPS

The acquisition of psychoacoustic and sensorimotor skills at an early age, for example, learning Beethoven, sets up complex, dedicated, and sensitive neural networks that actively proliferate and prune as a musician develops in his education from student to professional (Zatorre & Peretz, 2001). There is a high risk of allostatic overload during this time because of the extreme demands for perfection in music education and competitive structure of the arts, production, and entertainment business.

This implies that a professional musician has a significant cumulative sound exposure and ergonomic stress even before entering the performing arts work-

places and may have already suffered significant hearing loss and repetitive strain injuries. The experience of the Musicians' Clinics of Canada only echoes this rather startling fact that 9 out of 10 musicians who present with work-related musculoskeletal disorders also have measurable hearing loss.

From a neurobiological perspective, injury at such an early age can be catastrophic to talented musicians hoping for a career in the future. And furthermore, these maladaptive changes in body maps are memorized in the areas of the brain, promoting interoceptive kindling of the psychoacoustic, sensorimotor, and emotional processing (Blakeslee & Blakeslee, 2007).

The traditional labor-management model of prevention does not necessarily apply to hearing loss and repetitive strain injuries among musicians, as the problem has often developed prior to participation in the music business. Opportunities for prevention lie in understanding the development of the performing artist at an early age, and the likelihood of success of these interventions predates the venues associated with professional employment.

KEY POINT

The traditional labor-management model of prevention does not necessarily apply to hearing loss, as the problem has often developed prior to participation in the music business.

CREATIVITY AND COCHLEA

Because of recent economic changes in the arts, production, and entertainment industry, self-employed individuals working in small- to medium-sized workgroups tend to be the rule. Gone are the days of large-scale salaried orchestra members as has been the tradition in North America and Europe. With the advent of electronic technology and the rapid dissemination of entertainment medium through video, compact discs, and the Internet, the creative process of making music and distributing musical art to audiences around the world has changed dramatically.

Music education takes place in schools, stores, living rooms, and basements and then in colleges and universities, exposing the musician to various risky environments. Yet much of the music making is done in studios, clubs, and concert venues that pose different sorts of risks. The student musician risks are influenced by the teacher and curriculum, whereas the professional musician risks are influenced largely by business variables.

Although the clinician has sophisticated techniques to assess and treat cochlear damage, the risk to the individual artist is controlled largely by the intrinsic drive to achieve creative excellence. The cumulative exposure to acoustic and ergonomic stressors increases only if the teacher, school, and business fuel this drive without protecting the musician from these risks. This drive to create in itself puts the musician at risk to deleterious changes in neuroplasticity that are extremely difficult to reverse (Andreasen, 2005).

Herein lies the challenge to apply the preventive interventions that currently exist. A clinic-based model whereby individual musicians choose a comprehensive health evaluation for musculoskeletal problems, performance anxiety, and hearing assessment is amenable to a multidisciplinary preventive approach.

In our clinical experience, many vocalists and instrumentalists are keenly aware of and interested enough in their performance abilities to implement strategies to optimize their human performance and prevent injury. Unfortunately, at the time of assessment, significant impairments affecting their ability to perform have already occurred.

KEY POINT

A clinic-based model whereby individual musicians choose a comprehensive health evaluation for musculoskeletal problems, performance anxiety, and hearing assessment are amenable to a multidisciplinary preventative approach.

DISTORTION AND DYSTONIA

The neurotoxicity from the allostatic overload on the developing auditory, somatosensory, and emotional neural networks of musicians results in a fusion and blurring of the receptive neural fields of musical processing (Altenmueller, 2006). Occupational health problems such as myofascial pain, anxiety, depression, nerve entrapments, and stress-related disorders are the direct result of the chronic overexposure to stress hormones such as cortisol.

The devastating impact of auditory distortion and loss of sensorimotor control is seen on a day-to-day basis in the musicians' clinic. The psychological toll on the musician is profoundly traumatic and often leads to life-threatening depression and addiction. Because music education and the music business have been described as one of occupational Darwinism or "survival of the fittest," the injured musician involved in a long and challenging process of rehabilitation is often left behind or just replaced. This unforgiving reality leads to shattered dreams and lifelong suffering.

There still exists a significant culture of denial in the arts community, especially at the level of educational institutions and music business management. Many symphony orchestras around the world are still in conflict over basic occupational health and safety measures to protect musicians from acoustic, ergonomic, and psychological trauma. Educational administrations tend to treat these injuries as excuses to avoid exams and performance juries rather than sentinel health events requiring rapid, effective interventions. The culture of "no pain, no gain" is still the rule among music students.

The courage of some professional musicians to speak out about their injuries and the tragic consequences to their musical performance and careers is a recent phenomenon. This can only increase awareness of the requirement for preventive interventions at many levels in the arts community, and changes in attitude are occurring because of these advocacy efforts.

KEY POINT

The music business has been described as one of occupational Darwinism, or survival of the fittest.

The mirror neurons of the clinician need to be empathetically tuned to the unique nature of these injuries and consequences to the artistic mind and body. Only then can a therapeutic alliance be created on an individual and a collective basis targeted at making changes from a neuroplasticity perspective (Doidge, 2007).

EVOLUTION AND EDUCATION

The connection between sound and emotion has been systematically investigated, questioning the role of music in evolution and why for thousands of years humans have been obsessed with creating and performing music (Levitin, 2006). This is the conceptual point of departure from the known effects of noise upon hearing to questioning why humans would expose themselves to music that could be harmful to their health. The surge of dopamine, a neurotransmitter, released in the nucleus accumbens and ventral tegmental area of the brain, gives rise to the pleasurable reaction stimulated by musical processing in the frontal and temporal lobes, somatosensory areas, limbic system, and cerebellar neural networks.

Educational efforts have been carried out in some conservatories and faculties of music and have had some degree of acceptance. At the level of elementary and secondary music programs, music teachers employed by school boards and private music schools have taken an active role in educating their students about these injuries and hearing loss. The resistance to implementation of preventive interventions is rooted in archaic pedagogical methodology originating in the European classical music of the last few hundred years. Possibly the only path to educational progress is sadly one of attrition rather than enlightenment.

The young musicians at risk of hearing loss are not only exposed at school and at home practice but also bombarded from various multimedia devices with headphones and speakers all day and throughout the night. The addictive nature of music is the ultimate challenge for a health professional. To protect the hearing of a population so heavily influenced by peer pressure and music business promotion will take more than educational efforts.

Organizations such as Hearing Education and Awareness for Rockers (HEAR) and the Canadian Foundation for Health in the Arts are nonprofit organizations with the mission of sensitizing performing artists to the issue of hearing loss and other performing arts–related hazards. These organizations have become crucial in the educational network by disseminating information to arts organizations such as orchestras, smaller musical groups, and teacher associations.

The role of instrument manufacturers and the entertainment industry has yet to join this educational effort. These corporate interests must begin to collaborate with the arts community and fund these educational efforts. This is not unlike the tobacco industry funding antismoking campaigns, and social change will likely come with similar difficulty.

The role of government and regulatory agencies in the prevention of noise induced hearing loss has been the topic of much scientific and political debate. Traditional efforts have been directed towards hearing conservation programs rather than reducing exposures at the source. Exposure reduction has been largely avoided, using economic nonfeasibility as the reason. Legislative changes in noise regulations have been systematically resisted by strong economic interests.

This is still common in the arts, production, and entertainment industry, and therefore targeting music education is more practical at this time. Comprehensive courses in occupational health and safety for music students at the college and university levels have recently been developed and implemented. Hopefully, this trend will continue and become a mandatory criterion for certification and funding at an institutional level.

FITNESS AND FEEDBACK

The concept of the musician as an "acoustic athlete" holds promise as a prevention strategy. There is now an increasing trend of accepting the human performance model for a number of reasons. In the world of professional sports, there is clear benefit demonstrated related to injury prevention and optimal performance. Although the immediate impact of devices such as custom molded in-the-ear monitors cannot be realized from a health perspective, the benefits to musical performance are, in contrast, readily perceived and appreciated.

This unique opportunity can be seized upon by the clinician to capture the attention of the musician and secondarily adopt healthy behaviors (Begley, 2007). The fact that performers of wide acclaim are starting to change their lifestyle by improving diet, exercise, and fitness sets an excellent example for the younger musician. Yet at an institutional and industry level, these values regarding health promotion fall upon deaf ears and closed minds.

KEY POINT

The concept of the musician as an acoustic athlete holds promise as a prevention strategy.

Recent neurobiological evidence shows that training your mind can change your brain through innovative therapeutic techniques such as neurofeedback and biofeedback. Many influential athletes and a few musicians have expressed benefits in health and well-being utilizing these types of therapy, as well as the positive impact on their careers. Daily practice of yoga, Pilates, tai chi, and meditation are well-established stress reduction techniques derived from Eastern healing traditions.

The education of physicians, nurses, and therapists has unfortunately been weak in the discipline of occupational health and safety. The economics of health care have favored an expensive illness treatment system and now created a health care funding crisis limiting access to medically necessary services. Prevention and health promotion have largely been ignored by government agencies and the insurance industry.

This only adds further pressure on health professionals to become aware and educate themselves on how to intervene in a timely and cost-effective manner. The development of arts medicine clinics across North America and Europe offers the opportunity for health professionals to practice this craft and hopefully stem the tide of these health problems in the arts, production, and entertainment industry.

GENIUS AND GOD

How Beethoven created great works of musical art while suffering from severe hearing loss draws attention to his tremendous drive to overcome this health problem (Mai, 2007). His musical genius has inspired generations of musicians to challenge the boundaries of established artistic tradition and also the current status quo of social and political mediocrity. Although he had recurrent bouts of severe depression and indulged in wine fortified with lead oxide, Beethoven produced over 120 hours of music that continue to be performed daily around the world. This leads to the question of what drives humans to create and perform music even

with the significant risks of illness and injury. The spiritual brain and the need for emotional and social connection are vital to the survival of the human species (Beauregard & O'Leary, 2007).

The discipline of arts medicine is still in its infancy, and the problem of hearing loss among musicians is a priority health problem. Practical strategies of intervening with a human performance prevention model offer the arts medicine clinician an important role in identifying and preventing this health problem. By incorporating the new knowledge presented in this chapter, standards and guidelines can be developed, to be disseminated through the arts community in a systematic and organized fashion.

The beneficiaries of these efforts—the young developing musicians—can learn and perform their music without these devastating injuries and in turn influence their students in the future to adopt a human performance prevention model. The soul of musicians to express their emotions about themselves and the world will continue regardless of the challenges presented from a health or economic perspective. The techniques and strategies offered by health professionals can hopefully reduce the allostatic overload inherent in this artistic pursuit.

SUMMARY

The natural history of sound exposure in a musician's career begins usually at an early age, often paralleling that of the development of speech and language skills. Enhancement of musical performance skills often accelerates to peak performance in early childhood and adolescence. This is in sharp contrast to the average industrial worker who takes on a job in his 20s and changes very little after that time.

The professional musician has a significant cumulative sound exposure and ergonomic stress even before entering the performing arts workplaces and may have already suffered significant hearing loss and repetitive strain injuries. The traditional labor-management model of prevention does not necessarily apply to hearing loss and repetitive strain injuries among musicians, as the problem has often developed prior to participation in the music business. A clinic-based model whereby individual musicians choose a comprehensive health evaluation for musculoskeletal problems, performance anxiety, and hearing assessment is amenable to a multidisciplinary preventative approach.

The discipline of arts medicine is still in its infancy, and the problem of hearing loss among musicians is a priority health problem. Practical strategies of intervening with a human performance prevention model offer the arts medicine clinician an important role in identifying and preventing this health problem.

REFERENCES

Altenmueller, E. (Ed.). (2006). *Music, motor control, and the brain*. Oxford, UK: Oxford University Press.

Andreasen, N. C. (2005). *The creating brain: The neuroscience of genius*. Washington, DC: Dana Press.

Beauregard, M., & O'Leary, D. (2007). *The spiritual brain: A neuroscientist's case for the existence of the soul*. Old Saybrook, CT: Tantor Media.

Begley, S. (2007). *Train your mind, change your brain: How a new science reveals our extraordinary potential to transform ourselves*. New York: Random House.

Blakeslee, S., & Blakeslee, M. (2007). *The body has a mind of its own: How body maps in your brain help you do (almost) everything better*. New York: Random House.

Doidge, N. (2007). *The brain that changes itself: Stories of personal triumph from the frontiers of brain science*. New York: Viking Press.

Levitin, D. J. (2006). *This is your brain on music: The science of a human obsession*. New York: Dutton.

Mai, F. M. (2007). *Diagnosing genius: The life and death of Beethoven*. Montreal, Canada: McGill-Queen's University Press.

Sapolsky, R. M. (2004). *Why zebras don't get ulcers* (3rd ed.). New York: Henry Holt and Company.

van der Kolk, B. A., & McFarlane, A. C. (2006). *Traumatic stress: The effects of overwhelming experience on mind, body, and society*. New York: The Guilford Press.

Zatorre, R. J., & Peretz, I. (2001). The biological foundations of music. *Annals of the New York Academy of Sciences, 930*, 1–462.

14 Towards a Functional Hearing Test for Musicians: The Probe Tone Method

BY FRANK A. RUSSO

The relationship between hearing outcomes in the real world and hearing thresholds obtained by pure-tone audiometry has long been recognized as weak (Davis, 1947; Hirsch, 1952). This fact presents a problem for hearing aid fitting and will continue to do so as long as people wish to use hearing in their day-to-day living. Over the last few decades, the problem has been alleviated to some extent by what have come to be known as functional hearing tests. Generally, these tests assess some aspect of real-world hearing (e.g., speech perception) under simulated real-world conditions (e.g., noisy environments). Examples of such tests include the SPIN-R (Bilger, Nuetzel, Rabinowitz, & Rzeczkowski, 1984; Kalikow, Stevens, & Elliot, 1977) and HINT tests (Nilsson, Soli, & Sullivan, 1994). In both tests, the procedure involves having the participant repeat back words presented in a background of noise. Word identification accuracy can be used to differentiate individuals who would otherwise be judged equivalent on the basis of pure-tone audiometry alone (Pichora-Fuller, Schneider, & Daneman, 1995). Thresholds obtained from pure-tone audiometry may also be inadequate for predicting hearing outcomes in the real world of musicians.

Although functional aspects of hearing can and probably should be discussed informally during a fitting, there may be additional benefit obtained from the administration of formal tests that have been designed to address functional aspects of hearing for musicians. The benefit of formal tests is potentially very high when one considers the paucity of theory and evidence regarding optimization of hearing aids for music (Chasin & Russo, 2004). In short, it appears that there is a need for the development of new tests for measurement of functional hearing in musicians. These functional tests for musicians could be incorporated into the fitting protocol as a supplement to more informal methods.

KEY POINT

There is a need for the development of new tests for measurement of functional hearing in musicians.

WHAT EXACTLY CONSTITUTES FUNCTIONAL HEARING FOR MUSICIANS?

A working definition of functional hearing in musicians is simply the extent to which the hearing faculty may be used to support music production. The assessment of functional hearing will thus depend in part on the type of music that will be performed. For example, for musicians performing in a multipart group (such as a string quartet), they should be able to monitor their performance while remaining aware of what the other players are doing. For musicians producing music on a non–fixed-pitch instrument (e.g., violin), they should be able to hear slight intonation problems. For musicians who play an instrument with timbre that can be shaped (such as voice), they should be able to hear as much of the spectrum as possible. These challenges are not mutually exclusive and with a suboptimal capacity for hearing, can easily add up to drain the cognitive resources of the performer. These same cognitive resources might otherwise be allocated towards expressivity and communication with the audience.

Regardless of the particular performance challenges a musician is faced with, one aspect of functional hearing that is almost always required is sensitivity to tonality. Tonality refers to the hierarchical organization of pitches around the tonic or key-note of a piece. In Western music, this organization has been described as a four-level hierarchy of stability. The highest stability is assigned to the tonic tone (do), followed by nontonic triad tones (mi, so), followed by nontriadic tones (re, fa, la, ti), and finally the nonscale tones. Although this hierarchy tends to be most

evident in classical music, it can be found in all genres of Western music including folk, pop, country, and punk. Across these different genres, pitches that occupy more stable positions in the hierarchy are more likely to start and end a piece and to occur more frequently. Tonal organization is interpreted and may be clarified by the musician through performance expression (Thompson & Cuddy, 1997). Beyond clarifying the overall structure of a piece, tonality is a determinant of tension (Smith & Cuddy, 2003), which is another critical aspect of performance expression. The process of interpreting and clarifying tonal organization is particularly important for music involving improvisation and/or frequent modulations between keys.

KEY POINT

One aspect of functional hearing that is almost always required is sensitivity to tonality.

PROBE TONE METHOD

The probe tone method can be used to quantify the psychological representation of tonality (Krumhansl & Shepard, 1979). In this method, the listener is provided with a key-defining context (e.g., a tone sequence based on the major triad) followed by a probe tone. On separate trials, a probe tone is drawn from each of the chromatic scale steps. The listener is asked to evaluate the extent to which each probe tone fits the context, normally on a seven-point scale that ranges from "fits very poorly" to "fits very well." The set of probe tone ratings forms the probe tone profile, which may be compared to a standardized profile. This comparison forms the basis of the proposed functional test of hearing for musicians.

The standardized profiles were derived from average probe tone ratings obtained across musically trained listeners and across a variety of key-defining contexts (Krumhansl & Kessler, 1982). They are consistent with music-theoretic descriptions of tonal stability and they may be used as a referent against which sensitivity to tonality may be estimated (Russo, Cuddy, Galembo, & Thompson, 2007). The strength of the correlation between a listener's probe tone ratings and the standardized profile is known as the recovery score and is reflective of the listener's sensitivity to tonality under a particular set of listening conditions.

Researchers in music cognition have used the probe tone method in order to study variability in sensitivity to tonality due to age (Halpern, Kwak, Bartlett, & Dowling, 1996; Minghella, Russo, & Pichora-Fuller, 2007), frequency range (Russo et al., 2007), and timbre (Cuddy, Russo & Galembo, 2007; Minghella et al., 2007). Although most listeners with healthy hearing will show sensitivity to the hierarchy of pitches implied by a key-defining sequence presented under ideal listening conditions, minor perturbations in the fine temporal structure of tones (e.g., inharmonicity) can lead to a significant loss in sensitivity to the tonal hierarchy—that is, lower recovery scores (Cuddy et al., 2007; Minghella et al., 2007). These perturbations are introduced naturally in tones produced by stringed

instruments due to deviations from ideal elasticity (Galembo, Askenfelt, Cuddy, & Russo, 2001; Russo et al., 2007). Similar perturbations may be introduced by an impaired auditory system (Schneider & Pichora-Fuller, 2001) or theoretically by the hearing aid itself.

KEY POINT

Researchers in music cognition have used the probe tone method in order to study variability in sensitivity to tonality due to age, frequency range, and timbre, and it may have some applicability to the assessment of musicians.

HOW TO ASSESS FUNCTIONAL HEARING IN MUSICIANS

In order to implement the proposed test in a hearing clinic, it is advisable to have MIDI software that will allow you to encode and play back melodies. The playback feature should allow for specification of the playback instrument so that the test tones can be customized in accord with your client's principal instrument. There are free software programs available that have this capability.[1]

The test should be administered in blocks of trials, where each block involves a particular configuration of hearing aid settings. The ideal playback level should be adjusted so that the test tones are equivalent to the unaided threshold.[2]

---

[1] e.g., Anvil

[2] The tones are presented at the unaided threshold so as to present a challenging listening situation. In this test, musicians are not responsible for performance and are thus able to recruit relatively more resources than would be possible in a performance situation.

Each block includes 12 trials, consisting of one presentation each of all of the chromatic scale steps (in random order of presentation). Each trial consists of a key-defining melodic context (do-mi-do-so) followed by a probe tone after a 1-second rest. The exact transposition of the key-defining context does not matter, so long as it is major (which results in more consistent responding than the minor) and within the normal pitch range of the musician's instrument. Notation of example probe tone trials is provided in Figure 14–1 and Figure 14–2. The probe tone in Figure 14–1 fits reasonably well with the key-defining context, whereas the probe tone in Figure 14–2 does not.

KEY POINT

In the probe tone method the recovery score is reflective of the listener's sensitivity to tonality under a particular set of listening conditions.

Interpreting the Results

The recovery score for a particular block is simply the correlation between the ratings and the standardized profile.[3] An example has been depicted in Table 14–1. Higher recovery scores indicate more sensitivity to tonality. The minimum recovery score is −1 and the maximum recovery score is +1. An acceptable recovery score for a musician would be .6 or greater.

The recovery scores for the example provided in Table 14–1 are .57 and .89 for the first and second settings, respectively. Further insights may be obtained by examining the pattern of probe tone ratings. In the example, the level of differentiation in stability ratings between tones for the first setting is quite poor and there seems to be a strong influence of pitch proximity from the tonic (i.e., stability ratings decreasing with greater pitch distance from tonic). Similar patterns of probe tone ratings have been observed in ratings obtained with pure

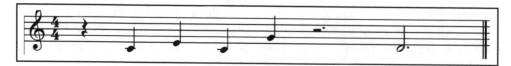

Figure 14–1. In this example of a probe tone trial, the key-defining context (do-mi-do-so) is followed by a probe tone (re) that fits reasonably well (i.e., a nontriadic scale tone).

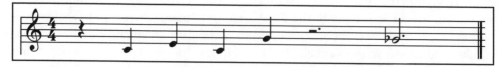

Figure 14–2. In this example of a probe tone trial, the key-defining context (do-mi-do-so) is followed by a probe tone (so-flat) that does not fit well (i.e., a nonscale tone).

---

[3]The standardized ratings are for the major mode and may thus be assigned to any major scale. For example, the standardized rating for G in G major would be equivalent to the standardized rating for C in C major (6.35).

Table 14–1. An example worksheet for a functional test of hearing for musicians based on the probe tone method

Client: Miles Davis

Playback instrument: Trumpet

Key/Tonic (do): C Major / C3

Hearing Aid Setting I: Parameter A: XX, Parameter B: XX, Parameter C: XX

Hearing Aid Setting II: Parameter A: XX, Parameter B: XX, Parameter C: XX

Scale Step	Ratings First Setting	Ratings Second Setting	Standardized Profile
C	5	7	6.35
C#	4	2	2.23
D	4	4	3.48
D#	3	3	2.33
E	3	5	4.38
F	3	4	4.09
F#	3	2	2.52
G	4	4	5.19
G#	3	2	2.39
A	3	5	3.66
A#	2	3	2.29
B	1	3	2.88
Recovery	**.57**	**.89**	

tones or with complex musical tones presented under adverse acoustic conditions (Cuddy et al., 2007).

Test Materials and Considerations for Testing

Blocked stimuli files (MIDI, WAVE, MP3), response keys, and additional instructions are available from the author's Web site (http://www.ryerson.ca/smart/func tional.html). As mentioned above, MIDI has the advantage of enabling customization (instrument and range). Nonetheless, the WAVE and MP3 files (realized with midrange piano tones) will give a reasonable indication of functional hearing and can be played using any media player.

If the performer is not a soloist, it may be advisable to perform the procedure with a background of pink noise. The spectral envelope of the pink noise is comparable to the long-term average spectrum of music, and may be useful in simulating the streaming demands placed upon the performing musician. Regardless of whether the pink noise manipulation is used, measurement error can be reduced by using multiple blocks for a setting (ratings across blocks can be averaged) and by providing a few practice trials in anticipation of any block.

GOING FORWARD: FORMALIZING THE PROPOSED TEST AND DEVELOPING OTHERS

An important aspect in the development of functional tests of hearing for speech has been the standardization process. In developing a functional hearing test for musicians, it would be ideal to aim for a similar level of rigor.

First, there is a need to demonstrate psychometric equivalence across different blocks (i.e., probe tone orderings) of the same test. This first issue may be broken down into a number of sub goals: (a) ensuring that different blocks of the same test are of equal difficulty; (b) ensuring that different blocks of the same test lead to homogeneity of variance; and (c) ensuring that the test is reliable such that measurements across multiple blocks of the same condition (e.g., same instrument and same settings) lead to comparable outcomes. In addition to the issue of equivalence across blocks, it would also be useful to establish test norms using representative samples so that an individual's hearing ability may be evaluated with respect to a particular population (compared with other people who play the same instrument).

Finally, as mentioned above, tonality is only one aspect of functional hearing in musicians, albeit ubiquitous in most genres of music. It would be useful to develop other functional tests that measure hearing skills that may be required for successful performance in specific genres of music (e.g., intonation tests for singers).

SUMMARY

A framework has been presented for administering a functional test of hearing for musicians. The test provides a measure of tonal sensitivity, which is an essential component of most music that is performed today. The framework can and should be customized to suit the needs of the individual performer. Although the functional test described has not been subjected to a standardization process, it seems reasonable to expect that it can be used on multiple occasions with the same client, thus providing a source of objective comparison of functional hearing obtained with different hearing aid settings.

REFERENCES

Bilger, R. C., Nuetzel, J. M., Rabinowitz, W. M., & Rzeczkowski, C. (1984). Standardization of a test of speech perception in noise. *Journal of Speech and Hearing Research*, *27*, 32–48.

Chasin, M., & Russo, F. A. (2004). Hearing aids and music. *Trends in Amplification*, *8*, 35–47.

Cuddy, L. L., Russo, F. A., & Galembo, A. (2007). Tonality of low-frequency synthesized piano tones. *Archives of Acoustics*, *32*, 541–550.

Davis, H. (1947). Hearing aids. In H. Davis (Ed.), *Hearing and deafness: A guide for laymen* (pp.161-210). New York: Murray Hill Books.

Galembo, A., Askenfelt, A., Cuddy, L. L., & Russo, F. A. (2001). Effects of relative phases on pitch and timbre in the piano bass range. *Journal of the Acoustical Society of America, 110*, 1649-1666.

Halpern, A. R., Kwak, S., Bartlett, J. C., & Dowling, W. J. (1996). Effects of aging and musical experience on the representation of tonal hierarchies. *Psychology and Aging, 11*, 235-246.

Hirsch, I. J. (1952). *The measurement of hearing*. New York: McGraw-Hill.

Kalikow, D. N., Stevens, K. N., & Elliot, L. L. (1977). Development of a speech intelligibility in noise using sentence materials with controlled word predictability. *Journal of the Acoustical Society of America, 61*, 1337-1351.

Krumhansl, C. L., & Kessler, E. J. (1982). Tracing the dynamic changes in perceived tonal organization in a spatial representation of musical keys. *Psychological Review, 89*, 334-368.

Krumhansl, C. L., & Shepard, R. N. (1979). Quantification of the hierarchy of tonal functions within a diatonic context. *Journal of Experimental Psychology: Human Perception and Performance, 5*, 579-594.

Minghella, D., Russo, F. A., & Pichora-Fuller, M. K. (2007). Effect of age on sensitivity to tonality. Proceedings of Acoustics Week in Canada. *Canadian Acoustics, 35*, 58-59.

Nilsson, M., Soli, S. D., & Sullivan, J. A. (1994). Development of the hearing in noise test for the measurement of speech reception thresholds in quiet and in noise. *Journal of the Acoustical Society of America, 95*, 1085-1099.

Pichora-Fuller, M. K., Schneider, B. A., & Daneman, M. (1995). How young and old adults listen to and remember speech in noise. *Journal of the Acoustical Society of America, 97*, 593-608.

Russo, F. A., Cuddy, L. L., Galembo, A., & Thompson, W. F. (2007). Variability in recovery of the tonal hierarchy across the pitch range. *Perception, 36*, 781-790.

Schneider, B. A., & Pichora-Fuller, M. K. (2001). Age-related changes in temporal processing: Implications for speech perception. *Seminars in Hearing, 22*, 227-239.

Smith, N. A., & Cuddy, L. L. (2003). Perceptions of musical dimensions in Beethoven's Waldstein Sonata: An application of Tonal Pitch Space Theory. *Musicae Scientiae, 7*, 7-31.

Thompson, W. F., & Cuddy, L. L. (1997). Music performance and the perception of key. *Journal of Experimental Psychology: Human Perception and Performance, 23*, 116-135.

Musical Note to Frequency Conversion Chart

A_0			A_3	110		A_6	880
B_0			B_3	123		B_6	988
C_0	16		C_3	131		C_6	1047
D_0	18		D_3	147		D_6	1175
E_0	21		E_3	165		E_6	1319
F_0	22		F_3	175		F_6	1397
G_0	25		G_3	196		G_6	1568
A_1	28		A_4	220		A_7	1760
B_1	31		B_4	247		B_7	1976
C_1	33		C_4	262		C_7	2093
D_1	37		D_4	294		D_7	2349
E_1	41		E_4	330		E_7	2637
F_1	44		F_4	349		F_7	2794
G_1	49		G_4	392		G_7	3136
A_2	55		A_5	440		A_8	3520
B_2	62		B_5	494		B_8	3951
C_2	65		C_5	523		C_8	4186
D_2	73		D_5	587		D_8	4699
E_2	82		E_5	659		E_8	5274
F_2	87		F_5	698		F_8	5588
G_2	98		G_5	784		G_8	6272

Conversion chart from letter note to frequency (Hz). Middle C on the piano keyboard is C_4 at 262 Hz, and the highest note on the piano is C_8 at 4186 Hz. Hearing is typically tested between C_4 and an octave above the highest note on the piano keyboard. A common notation is to have both the note and the frequency together, as A[440], which is also A_5. To get the semitone frequency, multiply the note below it by $^{12}\sqrt{2}$ or 1.0595. *Note.* From *The Acoustical Foundations of Music* (p. 153), by J. Backus, 1977, New York: W. W. Norton & Company, Inc. Copyright 1977 by W. W. Norton & Company, Inc. Adapted with permission.

Six Musicians' Fact Sheets

EDITOR'S NOTE

These sheets are written at the level of the musician and are summaries of some of the strategies and technologies that can allow musicians to hear and play their music safely. They have been used at the Musicians' Clinics of Canada for almost 20 years and can be found at our Web site at http://www.musiciansclinics.com. They can be photocopied and are free to anyone for use.

GUITAR AND ROCK/BLUES VOCALISTS

Guitar players and rock/blues vocalists share a similar part of the stage and, as such, are similarly exposed to loud music. Some of the strategies to reduce the potential for music related hearing loss are also similar.

- Ear monitors are small in-the-ear devices that look like hearing aids connected to small wire cables. These can be plugged directly into the amplification system. These not only afford some protection from overly loud music, but allow the guitar players and vocalists to monitor their music better. Frequently, the overall sound levels on stage during rehearsals and performances are quieter while using these monitors. In the case of vocalists, the use of ear monitors will allow them to hear their voice better with an added benefit of reduced vocal strain after a long set. Ear monitors can be designed to either improve monitoring or function as ear protection, or both. Depending on the type of music, one's style, and one's position in the band, a trade-off between these goals may be necessary.
- Loudspeakers generate a wide range of sounds. Like the bell of a trumpet, however, not all sounds come directly out of the speaker. Low frequency bass notes can be just as loud beside the loudspeaker enclosure as directly in front, whereas higher frequency sounds emanate much like a laser beam. Tilting or aiming the loudspeaker up to the musicians' ear will ensure that the music has a "flatter" response. The overall level will tend to be lower on stage because the sound engineer will not need to compensate for a "peaky" response. Some researchers recommend elevating loudspeakers to ear level for much the same reason. Indeed, this can be useful, but this will depend on the design of the loudspeaker. Checking with the manufacturer will provide information on whether this is the best choice of orientation for that specific loudspeaker.
- The loudspeakers can also be used as an acoustic shadow to hide in. As stated above, high frequency sounds tend to emanate from the loudspeakers in almost a straight line. Since these same high frequency treble notes can also be the most intense, standing beside the loudspeaker enclosure (instead of in front or behind it) may afford some protection.
- The main source of potential damage appears to be from the drummer's high hat cymbal—typically on the left side of the drummer. Moving away from the high hat cymbal as much as is reasonable, or the use of Lucite or Plexiglas baffles between the cymbals and the other musicians, may be useful to minimize the potential damage to one's hearing. If baffles are used, it is important to ensure that they do not extend above the level of the drummer's ear, since high frequency reflections can exacerbate the drummer's hearing.
- There are now custom made tuned earplugs that many instrumental musicians and vocalists use called the ER-15 earplugs. These allow all of the music to be attenuated (lessened in energy) equally across the full range of musical sounds. That is, the low bass notes are treated identically to the mid-range and high frequency treble notes. The balance of music is therefore not altered. These have been in wide use since the late 1980s.
- The human ear is much like any other body part—too much use and it may be damaged. The ear takes about 16 hours to reset. After attending a rock concert or a loud session, you may notice reduced hearing and/or tinnitus (ringing) in your ears. And if your hearing was assessed immediately after the concert, one would find a temporary hearing loss. After 16 hours, however, your hearing should return to its "baseline" (hopefully normal) level. After a loud session or concert, don't practice for 16 to 18 hours. Also, it's a good excuse not to mow your lawn for a day or two!

WOODWINDS AND LARGE STRINGED INSTRUMENTS

Woodwinds such as clarinet, saxophone, oboe, bassoon, and the flute are all found in symphonies and smaller chamber groups. So are the larger stringed instruments such as cello, string bass, and the harp. These instruments generate similar sound levels (albeit at different frequencies), and are subject to similar music exposure from other instruments. Many of these musicians need to sit in front of potentially damaging trumpet and percussion sections.

- Most of these instruments possess significant low frequency sound energy with very little fundamental and harmonic energy in the higher frequencies. And these same musicians need to sit downwind of the brass section. Most of the damaging energy from the brass section is in the higher frequency ranges, so it would be ideal to have ear protection that lets through the lower frequency sounds but attenuates (or lessens) the higher frequencies from the other instruments. Indeed such a vented/tuned earplug is useful for these instruments. A tuned cavity is created in the earplug that allows the musician to hear her own instrument while ensuring that the damaging elements of the trumpet and percussion sections are reduced.

- For those woodwinds (clarinet, saxophone, flute) that also play in jazz and blues bands, a wider form of protection can be useful. These are called the ER-15 earplugs. They allow all of the music to be attenuated (lessened in energy) equally across the full range of musical sounds. That is, the low bass notes are treated identically to the mid-range and high frequency treble notes. The balance of music is therefore not altered. These earplugs have been in wide use since the late 1980s.

- Plexiglas baffles can be erected between the cymbals and the jazz/blues woodwind players, but should not extend higher than the drummer's ear. Such baffles can attenuate the sound energy of the drums for the other musicians. Not extending the baffles too high ensures that the drummer is not subject to her own high frequency reflections, which may increase the potential for future hearing loss.

- Ear monitors are small in-the-ear devices that look like hearing aids connected to small wire cables. They can be connected directly to the amplification system. These not only afford some protection from overly loud music, but allow the woodwind players to monitor their music better. Generally, however, these are not necessary unless the music levels are very intense. Frequently, the overall sound levels on stage during rehearsals and performances are quieter while using these ear monitors.

- Acoustic monitors are stethoscope-like devices that can be used by acoustic bass, cello, and harp players to allow them to better hear their own instrument. A length of hearing aid tubing plugs into one's custom made earplug on one end and, by way of a suction cup or similar attachment, it plugs onto the tailpiece, bridge, or body of the bass, cello, or harp. The musician can better monitor her own instrument, which has the benefit of not overplaying. Wrist and arm strain is usually reduced with such a setup.

- The human ear is much like any other body part—too much use and it may be damaged. The ear takes about 16 hours to reset. After attending a rock concert or a loud session you may notice reduced hearing and/or tinnitus (ringing) in your ears. And if your hearing was assessed immediately after the concert, you would find a temporary hearing loss. After 16 hours, however, your hearing should return to its baseline (hopefully normal) level. After a loud session or concert, don't practice for 16 to 18 hours. Also, it's a good excuse not to mow your lawn for a day or two!

BASS PLAYERS AND DRUMMERS

Even though it may be surprising, group bass players and drummers may experience similar types of noise exposure because of their similar location in a band. In some cases, the environmental strategies to minimize the potential of hearing loss are also similar.

- Humming just prior to and through a loud sound, such as a cymbal crash or rim shot, may afford some hearing protection. There is a small muscle in our middle ears that contracts upon the sensation of loud sounds. This contraction pulls on the bones of the middle ear, thus temporarily making it harder for sound to be transmitted through to one's inner ear. Mother nature designed us with this, so that our own voice would not be perceived as too loud. If you know about an imminent loud sound such as a cymbal crash, hum just before the crash and sustain the hum through the sound.

- Shakers are small, hockey puck-sized speakers that can be wired into the main amplification system. These shakers can be bolted under a drummer's seat or screwed onto a 1 square foot piece of $3/4$ inch plywood board placed on the floor near the bass player or drummer. The musicians feel they are playing slightly louder than they actually are. The musicians are happy and their ears are happy.

- Plexiglas baffles can be erected between the cymbals and the bass players, but should not extend higher than the drummer's ear. Such baffles can attenuate (lessen) the sound energy of the drums for the other musicians. Not extending the baffles too high ensures that the drummer is not subject to her own high frequency reflections, which may increase the potential for future hearing loss.

- Ear monitors are small in-the-ear devices that look like hearing aids connected to small wire cables. They can be plugged directly into to the amplification system. These not only afford some protection from overly loud music, but allow the bass players and drummers to monitor their music better. Frequently, the overall sound levels on stage during rehearsals and performances are quieter while using these monitors.

- Acoustic monitors are stethoscope-like devices that can be used by acoustic bass and cello players to allow them to better hear their own instrument. A length of thin hearing aid tubing plugs into one's custom made earplug on one end and, by way of a suction cup or similar attachment, it plugs onto the tailpiece, bridge, or body of the bass. The bass musician can better monitor her own instrument, which has the benefit of not overplaying. Wrist and arm strain is usually reduced with such a setup.

- Drummers should be using the ER-25 earplugs. Too much ear protection can and does result in arm and wrist strain (due to overplaying), and not enough protection can result in continued hearing loss. The ER-25 (like its more mild form, the ER-15) is a uniform or flat ear protector such that the bass notes, the mid-range notes, and the high frequency notes are all attenuated equally. The balance of music is not altered.

- The human ear is much like any other body part—too much use and it may be damaged. The ear takes about 16 hours to reset. After attending a rock concert you may notice reduced hearing and/or tinnitus (ringing) in your ears. And if your hearing was assessed immediately after the concert, you would find a temporary hearing loss. After 16 hours, however, your hearing should return to its baseline (hopefully normal) level. After a loud session or concert, don't practice for 16 to 18 hours. Also, it's a good excuse not to mow your lawn for a day or two!

SCHOOL BAND TEACHERS

Several inexpensive modifications can be made to school classrooms and portables. Such venues may not be optimal for use as music rooms. These modifications can be accomplished without any special technical knowledge. In addition, other modifications can be made by acoustical engineers. While this second option may be costly, many of the recommendations made by acoustical engineers may yield dramatically improved acoustic environments.

- Trumpets and other treble brass instruments should be placed on risers. Most of the damaging energy of the trumpet is in the higher frequency ranges, and these high frequency treble notes tend to emanate from the bell of the trumpet like a laser beam. That is, high frequency damaging sounds will tend to go over the heads of those other musicians downwind. In addition, the trumpet players will not need to play as hard for their sound to be heard clearly. And by the time the trumpet sound reaches the conductor, the levels are not nearly as damaging as for those immediately in front of the trumpets.

- A highly reflective surface, such as a blackboard, behind the teacher/conductor is the worst possible wall covering. High frequency sounds tend to reflect off such surfaces, thereby adding to the overall intensity level in the room. Moveable drapes or thick curtains can be hung over the blackboard (or concrete wall) to absorb these unwanted reflections. They can then be pulled aside when the blackboard is being used.

- Carpeting can be used at the front of the room where the conductor stands. Not only will this absorb some of the undesirable reflections, but will also allow the music teacher to stand for longer periods of time without backaches.

- Three-dimensional relief art (from the art department) would make an excellent wall covering for the side walls of the music room. In this location, the art will not be visually distracting and at the same time absorb many of the undesirable mid- and high frequency reflections.

- There are now custom made tuned earplugs that many musicians and music teachers are using called ER-15 earplugs. These allow all of the music to be attenuated (lessened in energy) equally across the full range of musical sounds. That is, the low bass notes are treated identically to the mid-range and high frequency treble notes. The balance of music is therefore not altered. These earplugs have been in wide use since the late 1980s.

- The human ear is much like any other body part—too much use and it may be damaged. The ear takes about 16 hours to reset. After attending a rock concert or a loud session at school you may notice reduced hearing and/or tinnitus (ringing) in your ears. And if your hearing was assessed immediately after the concert, you would find a temporary hearing loss. After 16 hours, however, your hearing should return to its baseline (hopefully normal) level. After a loud session or concert, don't practice for 16 to 18 hours. Also, it's a good excuse not to mow your lawn for a day or two!

VIOLINS AND VIOLAS

Violins and violas can generate sufficiently loud levels of music such that they can cause permanent hearing loss. This is typically worse in the left ear (the ear nearer the instrument). In many cases, the violin or viola player is surrounded by many like instruments, so that the overall level in the violin and viola sections of an orchestra can be quite intense. Unlike most other instrument categories, the ability to hear the higher frequency harmonics is crucial to these musicians. Therefore, recommendations are provided to protect hearing and to maintain audibility of the higher frequency harmonics.

■ Violins and violas should always be played away from overhangs such as those commonly found in orchestral pits. The roofs of such overhangs frequently are treated acoustically in order to minimize reflections. It is not uncommon that the magnitude of the higher frequency harmonic components of these instruments are reduced by this acoustic treatment. Since players of violins and violas need to be aware of this high frequency energy, the sound is muted. These musicians tend to play harder to compensate for this lost energy with an unnecessary increased sound level and a possible danger to their arms.

■ There are any number of acoustic baffles that can be placed on the rear portion of a seat in an orchestra that can serve to reduce the loudness of the instruments to the rear. Depending on the manufacturer, some are opaque and some are transparent. Baffles work well and serve to attenuate (or lessen) higher frequency sounds more than bass sounds. However, these seat baffles only work if the baffle is within 7 inches of the musician's ear. If further away, because of reflections off the floor and music stands, the baffles have no significant effect.

■ Like other instruments, violin and viola players can use mutes while practicing, thus reducing the overall daily exposure to noise/music. These mutes can fit over the bridge and only result in a slight loss of high frequency musical information.

■ There are now custom made tuned earplugs that many violin and viola players are using called ER-15 earplugs. These allow all of the music to be attenuated (lessened in energy) equally across the full range of musical sounds. That is, the low bass notes are treated identically to the mid-range and high frequency treble notes. The balance of music is therefore not altered. These earplugs have been in wide use since the late 1980s.

■ The human ear is much like any other body part—too much use and it may be damaged. The ear takes about 16 hours to reset. After attending a rock concert or a loud musical session, you may notice reduced hearing and/or tinnitus (ringing) in your ears. And if your hearing was assessed immediately after such a concert or session, you would find a temporary hearing loss. After 16 hours, however, your hearing should return to its baseline (hopefully normal) level. After a loud session or concert, don't practice for 16 to 18 hours. Also, it's a good excuse not to mow your lawn for a day or two!

HEARING LOSS PREVENTION FOR MUSICIANS— EARPLUGS, HUMMING, AND MODERATION

Hearing loss is a gradual process that may not be noticed for years. And when it does happen, people generally notice that speech is mumbled and unclear. People may report a ringing (or tinnitus) in their ears. By that time, it may be too late. Prevention of hearing loss is where it's at!

There are many sources of noise in the music industry—explosions, loud cymbal crashes, feedback from speakers, and the routine noise and music of a busy life. Yet even quiet noises, if one listens to them long enough, can damage one's hearing. A dial tone on a telephone, if listened to long enough, can cause a permanent hearing loss. It's not just rock music—it can be your Walkman, or even a symphony! A permanent hearing loss can be the result of a single loud blast, but more often it's the result of years of exposure to sounds that one would not normally think of as damaging.

Conventional hearing protection has historically not been well received by those in the performing arts and by music listeners. This form of foam plug usually causes the wearer to hear speech as if it was muffled and unclear. In addition, frequently one's own voice sounds hollow and echoey. There is a tuned earplug called the ER-15 earplug, and it treats all sound identically—the low bass notes, the mid-range, and the higher treble notes are all lessened or attenuated by the same 15 decibels. With this earplug, speech is clear and there is significant reduction of the potential for hearing loss from loud sounds. People who wear the ER-15 frequently forget that they are actually wearing ear protection.

Another strategy is to hum while you work. Humans (and all other mammals) have a small muscle in their middle ears that contracts upon loud sounds. From an evolutionary perspective, we have such a muscle so that our own voice will not be too loud for us. When this muscle (called the stapedius muscle) contracts, it pulls on the chain of bones in the ear that conducts sounds, making them less efficient as conductors. Sound from the environment therefore cannot get through to our ears as readily, thus providing us with significant protection. If you know that a loud sound or blast is about to occur, start humming before the blast and continue until the blast is finished. Drummers have known this for years without being told.

Finally, permanent hearing loss starts as a series of temporary hearing losses. When you come out of a rock concert or other loud venue, your hearing may temporarily be decreased. You might notice this as a muffled feeling and may notice ringing or tinnitus. This temporary hearing loss resolves after about 16 to 18 hours. Eventually it may become permanent. The strategy would therefore involve moderation. If you see a loud rock group on Friday night, don't mow your lawn on Saturday. Wait until Sunday, or better still, get someone else to do it!

Index

A

Absorptive wall panels, 94
ACE, 119
Acoustical glare, 87–88
"Acoustic athlete," 141–142
Acoustic bass, 3
Acoustic defects, 87–88, 96
Acoustic monitors, 157–158
Acoustics
    adequately intense performance sound
        level, 84–85
    background sound levels, 84–85
    design considerations, 90
    early first sound reflections, 85–87
    evenly distributed sound, 87–88
    music rehearsal spaces, 92–93
    practice rooms, 94
    reverberation time, 88–91, 96
    teaching rooms, 94
Acoustic tumor, 43
Aging induced hearing loss, 42–43
Air-conditioning systems, 85
All-or-none spike discharges, 23
Allostasis, 137–138
Allostatic overload, 138–139
Allowable daily exposures, 64
Aminoglycoside antibiotics, 35
Amphitheaters, 84
Amplified guitar, 3
Amplifiers
    bass settings on, 98–99
    elevation of, on stage, 100
Analog-to-digital converter, 109–110
Animal models, 2
Annoyance hyperacusis, 48–49
Apparent source width, 87

Arts medicine, 142
Attenuation, earplug effects on, 65–66
Attenuators, 67–68, 70
Audience
    loudspeaker monitoring systems' effect
        on, 76
    "miking" of, 79
    sound propagation to, 84
Audiologic assessment, 36
Audiologist, 79–80
Audiology, 129–130
Audiometric asymmetries, 7
Auditoriums
    background sound levels, 84–85
    design of, 88, 90
    diffuse sound field in, 88
    environmental modifications in. See
        Environmental modifications
    evenly distributed sound, 87–88
    orchestra pits, 93–94
    studies of, 83–84
    upholstered seats in, 88–90
Auditory nerve
    fiber responses of, 23–27
    output of, 27
Auditory pathway, 11–12
Auricle, 11–12

B

BabyBlues earplug, 72
Background noise, 98
Background sound, 84–85
Baffles, 84, 103–104, 156–158, 160
Band placement on stage, 101–102
Baroque sacred music, 90

Basilar membrane, 15, 18
Bass drum, 3
Bassoon, 2, 157
Bass players, 158
Beethoven, Ludwig von, 47, 142
Behind-the-ear hearing aids, 112–113, 131
Bimodal stimulation, 124
Binaural quality index, 87
Binaural summation, 81
Biofeedback, 141
Blues vocalists, 156
Body maps, 138
Boston Symphony Hall, 88–89

C

Canadian Foundation for Health in the
    Arts, 141
Carpeting, 159
Cassette tape players, 54–55
CD players, 54–56
Ceilings, 92, 94
Cello, 3
Central auditory pathway, 27
CHABA. *See* Committee on Hearing and
    Bioacoustics
Chamber music, 3
Characteristic frequency, 25
Chloride, 14
Clarinet, 2–3, 132, 134, 157
Click-evoked transient otoacoustic
    emissions, 22
Clouds, 84
Cochlea
    anatomy of, 12, 14–15
    damage to, 138–139
    inner hair cells, 16–17, 54, 118
    mechanics of, 18–20
    neural activity in, 11
    nonlinear behavior in, 20
    organ of Corti, 16
    otoacoustic emissions. *See* Otoacoustic
        emissions
    outer hair cells, 16–17, 36, 118
    pressure fluctuations in, 18
    transduction, 16–17
    traveling wave amplitude displacement,
        18–19

Cochlear implants
    acoustic hearing aids and, 125–126
    block diagram of, 118–119
    in children, 124
    early uses of, 117
    input systems, 118
    mechanism of action, 118–121
    music appraisal by recipients of,
        121–126
    music perception improvements,
        123–126
Cochlear nuclei, 27
Committee on Hearing and Bioacoustics
    damage risk criteria developed by, 4,
        6–7
    description of, 4
Concert halls
    adequately intense performance sound
        level, 84–85
    background sound levels, 84–85
    design of, 88, 90
    diffuse sound field in, 88
    environmental modifications in. *See*
        Environmental modifications
    evenly distributed sound, 87–88
    orchestra pits, 93–94
    reverberation time, 88–91, 96
    scale modeling of, 88
    sound reinforcement systems, 91–92
    studies of, 83–84
    upholstered seats in, 88–90
Cortisol, 139
Counseling, 44
Cranial nerve VIII. *See* Auditory nerve
Crest factors, 108
Cumulative sound exposure, 138, 143
Cymbals, 104, 156, 158

D

Damage risk criteria, 4, 6–7, 59, 64–65
Darwinism, occupational, 139–140
Deiters cell, 16
Desensitization, 38
DeVitto, Liberty, 46
Diffuse sound field, 88
Digital music players, 55–57, 59
Diplacusis, 34, 38

Directional microphones, 113
Distortion product otoacoustic emissions, 20, 22–23
Dopamine, 140
DRC. *See* Damage risk criteria
Drummers, 158
Dynamic range, 1–2, 26–27

E

Ear
  external, 11–13
  inner. *See* Cochlea
  middle, 12–14
Early decay time, 91
Early first sound reflections, 85–87
Earmuffs, 44
Earphones, for in-the-ear monitors, 77–79, 81
Earplugs
  attenuation imbalances caused by, 65–66
  custom-made, 156
  ER-15. *See* Musicians Earplugs™
  ER-20, 71–72
  ER-25, 158
  flat-response moderate attenuation, 63
  high fidelity. *See* High fidelity earplugs
  hyperacusis management using, 48
  limitations of, 65–66, 73
  noise reduction rating, 72–73
  non-custom, 71–72
  occlusion effect caused by, 66, 68
  recommendations for, 69
  tinnitus prevention, 44
Echo, 87
"Effective quiet," 4
Endolymph, 17
Endolymphatic space, 14
Environmental modifications
  baffles, 84, 103–104, 156–158, 160
  description of, 36
  instrument locations, 104
  monitoring improvements, 98–99
  orchestra/band should be set back from the edge of the stage, 101–102
  speaker/amplifier enclosures should be elevated, 100
  treble brass instruments placed on risers, 100–101, 159
  treble stringed instruments placed away from overhangs, 102
Environmental Protection Agency, 5
Equal loudness curves, 112
ER-15 earplug. *See* Musicians Earplugs™
ER-20 earplug, 71–72
ER-25 earplug, 158
Eustachian tube, 13
Exchange rates, 6
External auditory canal, 11–12
External ear
  anatomy of, 11–13
  sound amplification testing, 13
  sound pressure, 13

F

Fear hyperacusis, 48–49
Feedback, 114–115, 141
f_2/f_1 ratio, 22
5 dB exchange rate, 6, 64, 73
Flat-response moderate attenuation earplugs, 63
Fletcher-Munson curves, 112
Flute, 3, 133–134, 157
Flutter echo, 87
Formants, 132
Forte, 130
French horn, 2–3
Frequency, musical notes converted to, 153
Frequency-hopping artifact, 114
Front of house engineer, 75–76
Functional hearing, 146
Functional hearing tests
  administration of, 147–148
  description of, 145
  MIDI software for, 147
  probe tone method. *See* Probe tone method
  psychometric equivalence, 150
  pure-tone audiometry, 145
  results of, 148–149
  standardization of, 150
  test materials and considerations, 149–150
  types of, 145

G

Glutamate ototoxicity, 5
Greek amphitheaters, 84
Guitar players, 156

H

Hair cells, 16-17, 23, 118
Half wavelength resonators, 133, 135-136
Harmonic distortion, 110
Headphones
    with cassette players, 54-55
    with CD players, 55-56
    ear positioning of, 56-57
    evidence regarding, 58, 60
    hearing damage caused by, 58-59
    listening levels, 57-58
    noise induced hearing loss caused by, 54
    with portable digital music players,
        55-57, 59
    time-weighted average estimates, 59
    volume recommendations for, 56
Hearing
    functional, 146
    physiology of, 118
Hearing aids
    analog-to-digital converter, 109-110
    behind-the-ear, 112-113, 131
    channels for music, 113
    cochlear implants and, 125-126
    compression parameters for, 114
    directional microphone, 113
    feedback reduction systems, 114-115
    front-end distortion, 109-110
    multichannel, 113
    music program recommendations,
        115-116
    noise reduction systems, 115
    peak input limiting level in, 109-113
    in tinnitus patients, 45
    turn down or dampen the input,
        111-112
Hearing Education and Awareness for
    Rockers (HEAR), 141
Hearing loss. *See also* Music induced
    hearing loss; Noise induced hearing
    loss

age-induced, 42-43
    educating musicians about, 140-141
    factors that affect, 2, 4-5
    medications that cause, 34-35
    prevention of. *See* Prevention
    sensorineural, 112, 118
    symmetrical, 7
    temporary, 156-161
Hearing protection
    by humming, 158, 161
    prevalence of, 44
Hearing protection devices
    diplacusis treated with, 38
    earplugs. *See* Earplugs
Hearing tests, functional
    administration of, 147-148
    description of, 145
    MIDI software for, 147
    probe tone method. *See* Probe tone
        method
    psychometric equivalence, 150
    pure-tone audiometry, 145
    results of, 148-149
    standardization of, 150
    test materials and considerations,
        149-150
    types of, 145
Hensen cells, 16
High fidelity earplugs
    attenuators, 67-68, 70
    description of, 66-68
    earmold construction, 69-70
    fitting of, 70
    impression technique for, 68-69
    performance verification, 70-71
    recommendations for, 69
High fidelity music, 113
High frequency sounds, 101-102
High hat cymbals, 156
High school music rooms, 94
HINT tests, 145
Homeostasis, 137
Humming, 158, 161
HVAC systems, 85
Hyperacusis
    annoyance, 48-49
    definition of, 48
    description of, 33-34

fear, 48–49
loudness, 48–49
treatment of, 38

I

Incus, 12–13
Industrial noise
  audiogram findings, 7
  modulation rate of, 1–2
  music and, comparisons between, 1–2
  OSHA regulations for, 58
  permissible exposure limits for, 64–65
  prevalence of exposure to, 53
  spectral energy of, 1
  symmetrical hearing loss caused by, 7
  tinnitus caused by, 42
Inferior colliculus, 27
Inner ear. *See* Cochlea
Inner hair cells, 16–17, 23, 54, 118
In situ microphones with in-the-ear
    monitors, 79, 81
Instrumental music, 1
Instruments. *See also specific instrument*
  conical, 133
  description of, 2–3
  mechanical resonances, 134–135
  percussive, 2–3, 135
  as resonators. *See* Resonators
  treble brass, 100–101, 159
  treble brass instruments, 100–101
  treble stringed instruments, 102
  volume-related resonances, 134–135
  woodwinds, 157
Intensity, 97–98, 129–130
Interaural cross-correlation coefficient, 91
International Organization for
    Standardization
  11904-2, 55
  R-1999, 5
In-the-ear monitors
  audiologist's role, 79–80
  benefits of, 76–77, 156–157
  components of, 76, 78
  custom-made, 77–79, 99
  dynamic diaphragms, 79
  earphones for, 77–79
  floor monitor levels matched with, 80–81

illustration of, 78, 99
isolation feelings caused by, 79
minimal acceptable listening level
    using, 80–81
purpose of, 75
safe use of, 80–81
in situ microphones with, 79, 81
sound level checks, 80
speaker technology, 79
tips for, 81–82
vocalist use of, 156
woodwind musicians' use of, 157
Intimacy, 87

K

Keyboards, 3

L

Labor-management model of prevention,
    138, 143
Lateral fraction, 87
Lateral reflections, 87
Letters, 129–130
Listening environment, 57–58
Long-term music spectrum, 107–108
Loudness
  hyperacusis caused by, 48–49
  intensity and, comparison between,
    97–98
Loudspeakers
  elevation of, on stage, 100
  enclosures for, 101
  monitoring systems for, 75–76
  sound production by, 156

M

Malleus, 12–13
Meatus, 11
Mechanical resonances, 134–135
Medial geniculate body, 27
Medical history, 34–35
Medications
  hearing loss caused by, 34–35
  tinnitus caused by, 43
Ménière's disease, 34, 43

Mezzo forte, 130
Middle ear
    anatomy of, 12–13
    pressure amplification function of, 14
Middle-ear tinnitus, 41
Minimal acceptable listening level, 80–81
Monitor engineer, 76–77
Monitors/monitoring
    improvements in, 98–99
    in-the-ear. *See* In-the-ear monitors
MP-3 player, 3
Multichannel hearing aids, 113
Music
    cochlear implant recipients' listening
        to, 121–126
    consumption of, 54
    industrial noise and, comparisons
        between, 1–2
    long-term spectrum, 107–108
    notations used in, 129–130, 135
    sources of, 107
Music addiction, 54, 140
Musical hallucinations, 46
Musical notes, 129–130, 135, 153
Music cognition, 147
Music consumers, 53–54
Music education, 139–140
Music exposure
    rest periods between, 42–43
    tinnitus caused by, 42, 46–47
Musicians
    bass players, 158
    cumulative sound exposure, 138, 143
    drummers, 158
    functional hearing in, 146
    guitar players, 156
    music consumption by, 54
    rock/blues vocalists, 156
    symphony, 63, 140
    with tinnitus, 46–47
Musicians Earplugstrademark
    attenuators, 67–68, 70
    description of, 66–68, 161
    earmold construction, 69–70
    fitting of, 70
    impression technique for, 68–69
    performance verification, 70–71
    recommendations for, 69

    school band teachers' use of, 159
    violinists' use of, 160
    vocalist use of, 156
Music induced hearing loss
    description of, 32–33
    onset of, 60
    prevention of, 43
    in symphony musicians, 63
    tinnitus as early sign of, 45–46
    treatment of, 36–37
Music rehearsal spaces, 92–93
Music therapy, for tinnitus, 47

N

National Institute for Occupational Safety
    and Health, 5, 64–65, 68
Neurofeedback, 141
Neurons, in superior olivary complex, 27
9 dB attenuation, 103
Noise
    allowable daily exposures, 64
    background, 98
    continuous, 44
    industrial. *See* Industrial noise
    OSHA regulations for, 58
    permissible exposure limits, 64, 68
    prevalence of, 53
    tinnitus induced by, 42
Noise cancellation headphones, 44
Noise dose, 65
Noise induced hearing loss
    description of, 32–33
    government's role in preventing, 141
    headphones use as cause of, 54
    otoacoustic emissions for diagnosis of,
        36
    predisposing factors, 34–35
    psychological effects of, 139
    tinnitus secondary to, 33, 46
    treatment of, 36–37
Noise induced otologic damage
    diplacusis, 34, 38
    hyperacusis, 33–34
    music induced hearing loss, 32–33
    overview of, 31–32
    prevalence of, 31–32
    problems caused by, 32–33

tinnitus. *See* Tinnitus
vestibular dysfunction, 34
Noise reduction rating, 72–73, 94
Noise reduction systems, of hearing aids, 115
Non-custom earplugs, 71–72
Notations, 129–130, 135
Notch filtering, 114

O

Oboe, 3, 136, 157
Occlusion effect, 66, 68
Occupational Darwinism, 139–140
Occupational health and safety, 142
Occupational Safety and Health Administration
noise regulations, 58, 64
sound exposure limits, 95
workplace sound levels, 94–95
On-stage monitoring
in-the-ear monitor system for. *See* In-the-ear monitors
loudspeaker systems, 75–76
traditional methods of, 75–76
Orchestra pits, 93–94
Orchestra placement on stage, 101–102
Organ of Corti, 16
OSHA. *See* Occupational Safety and Health Administration
OSPL90, 108
Ossicles, 12–13
Otoacoustic emissions
definition of, 36
distortion product, 20, 22–23
noise induced hearing loss detection using, 36
spontaneous, 20–21
transient. *See* Transient otoacoustic emissions
Outer hair cells, 5, 16–17, 36, 118
Oval window, 13–14
Overhangs, 102, 160

P

Partial masking, 45, 47
Peak input limiting level, 109–113

Peak limiters, 81
Percussion, 2–3, 135
Performance sound levels, 84–85
Perilymph, 14
Permanent threshold shift
description of, 2, 4
manifestation of, 4
models of, 5–6
physiological mechanisms of, 5
studies of, 5–6
temporary threshold shift and, 8
Permissible exposure limits, 64, 68
Personal monitors. *See* In-the-ear monitors
Phase cancellation, 114
Phonemics, 109
Phonetics, 109
Physical examination, 35–36
Pianissimo, 130
Piano, 3
Piccolo, 3, 133
Pink noise, 149–150
Pitch, 122, 147
Platinum derivative antineoplastic agents, 35
Portable digital music players, 55–57, 59
Poststimulus time histogram, 25–26
Potassium, 17
Practice rooms, 94
Presbycusis, 42
Pressure amplification, 14
Prevention. *See also specific methods*
importance of, 140–141
labor-management model of, 138, 143
methods of, 36
Probe tone method
administration of, 147–148
examples of, 148
MIDI software for, 147
principles of, 146–147
results of, 148–149
standardized profiles, 147
test materials and considerations, 149–150
tonality sensitivity studies using, 147
Proscenium style theaters, 84
PTS. *See* Permanent threshold shift
Pure-tone audiometry, 145

Q

Quarter wavelength resonators, 131–133

R

Recruitment, 38
Reflections
  early first sound, 85–87
  lateral, 87
  law of, 89
Reflective ceiling, 92, 94
Reflective panels, 84
Rehearsal spaces, 92–93
Reissner's membrane, 14–15
Resistive network, 111
Resonators
  classification of, 130–131
  definition of, 130
  half wavelength, 133, 135–136
  quarter wavelength, 131–133
Reverberation time
  description of, 88–91
  in music rehearsal spaces, 92
Ring Cycle, 2, 108
Rock vocalists, 156
Roman amphitheaters, 84
Room acoustics
  adequately intense performance sound
    level, 84–85
  background sound levels, 84–85
  design considerations, 90
  early first sound reflections, 85–87
  evenly distributed sound, 87–88
  music rehearsal spaces, 92–93
  practice rooms, 94
  reverberation time, 88–91, 96
  teaching rooms, 94
Root mean square, 108
Round window membrane, 14

S

Saxophone, 3, 157
Scala media, 14–15
Scala vestibuli, 14–15
Scale modeling, 88
School band teachers, 159

Seat-dip effect, 88
Secular baroque music, 90
Sensorineural hearing loss, 112, 118
Sensorineural tinnitus, 41
Shakers, 158
Side-fills, 75
Singers. *See* Vocalists
6 dB attenuation, 103
Sleep disturbances, 41, 45
Smetana, Bedrich, 47
Smoking, 34
Sound
  emotion and, connection between,
    140
  evenly distributed, 87–88
  speed of, 87
Sound engineers, 75–76, 101
Sound exposure, 95, 137–138, 142
Sound field, diffuse, 88
Sound focusing, 88
Sound intensity, 97–98
Sound level meters, 43, 97
Sound levels, 44
Sound reflections, early first, 85–87
Sound reinforcement systems, 91–92
Sound therapy, 44–45
Source shift, 87
Speakers
  elevation of, on stage, 100
  enclosures for, 100
  sound production by, 156
Spectrogram, 120
Speech
  crest factors, 108
  long-term spectrum, 107
  phonetic vs. phonemic perceptual
    requirements, 109
Speech comprehension difficulties, 32
Speed of sound, 87
SPIN-R test, 145
Spiral ligament, 14–15
Spontaneous otoacoustic emissions,
  20–21
Stage
  instrument locations, 104
  orchestra/band placement on, 101–102
  speaker/amplifier enclosures elevated
    on, 100

treble brass instruments placed on risers, 100–101, 159
treble stringed instruments placed away from overhangs, 102
Standing waves, 87
Stapedius, 161
Stapes, 12–14, 18
Stereocilia, 16–18
Streisand, Barbara, 46
Stress hormones, 139
Stress reduction, 142
Stria vascularis, 14–15
Superior olivary complex, 27
Surface diffusivity index, 88
Symmetrical hearing loss, 7
Symphony musicians, 63, 140

T

Teaching rooms, 94
Temporary hearing loss, 156–161
Temporary threshold shift
   from cassette tape player volume, 55
   glutamate ototoxicity as cause of, 5
   manifestation of, 4
   permanent threshold shift and, 8
   physiological mechanisms of, 5
   resolution of, 2
   in rock music listeners, 32, 161
Texture of sound, 87
Thalamus, 27
3 dB attenuation, 103
3 dB exchange rate, 6, 64–65, 73
Time-weighted average estimates, 59
Tinnitus
   acoustic tumor and, 43
   aging and, 42–43
   causes of, 42–43
   definition of, 33, 41
   duration of, 2
   hearing aids for, 45
   hyperacusis and, 33
   industrial noise as cause of, 42
   medication-induced, 43
   Ménière's disease and, 43
   middle-ear, 41
   as music, 46
   music exposure and, 42

   musicians with, 46–47
   music induced hearing loss secondary to, 45–46
   music therapy for, 47
   noise exposure and, 42
   noise induced hearing loss and, 33, 46
   partial masking of, 45, 47
   prevalence of, 33, 44
   prevention of, 43–44
   risk groups for, 41–42
   self-help resources for, 45
   sensorineural, 41
   sleeping affected by, 41, 45
   songs about, 47–48
   sound therapy for, 44–45
   symptoms of, 41
   treatment of, 37–38, 44–46
Tinnitus Activities Therapy, 44
Tinnitus Handicap Inventory, 37
Tinnitus Retraining Therapy, 37–38
Tinnitus Severity Index, 37
Tonality, 146, 150
Townsend, Pete, 46
Transduction, 16–17
Transient otoacoustic emissions
   description of, 21–23
   headphone studies, 58–59
Traveling wave amplitude displacement, 18–19
Treble brass instruments, 100–101, 159
Treble clef, 130
Treble stringed instruments, 102
Trombone, 2–3
Trumpets, 2–3, 100–101, 104, 159
TTS. *See* Temporary threshold shift
Tuba, 2
Tympani, 3
Tympanic membrane, 11, 118

U

Upholstered seats, 84, 88–90

V

Venting of personal monitors, 81
Vestibular dysfunction, 34
Violas, 160

Violin, 2–3, 33, 160
Vocalists
    high frequency hearing loss effects on, 33
    in-the-ear monitor use by, 156
    rock, 156
Vocal music, 1
Volume-related resonances, 134–135

W

Wagner's Ring Cycle, 2, 108
Wedges, 75, 99
Wide dynamic range compression, 114
Woodwind instruments, 157